The traditional home doctor

Books by the same author include:

The Medicine Men (1975)
Paper Doctors (1976)
Everything You Want to Know About
   Ageing (1976)
Stress Control (1978)
The Home Pharmacy (1980)
Aspirin or Ambulance (1980)
Face Values (1981)
Guilt (1982)
The Good Medicine Guide (1982)
Stress and Your Stomach (1983)
Bodypower (1983)
Thomas Winsden's Cricketing Almanack
   (1983)
A Guide to Child Health (1984)
An A to Z of Women's Problems (1984)
Bodysense (1984)
Taking Care of Your Skin (1984)
Diary of a Cricket Lover (1984)
Life Without Tranquillisers (1985)
High Blood Pressure (1985)
Diabetes (1985)
Arthritis (1985)
Eczema and Dermatitis (1985)
The Story of Medicine (1985)
Natural Pain Control (1986)
Mindpower (1986)
Addicts and Addictions (1986)
Dr Vernon Coleman's Guide to
   Alternative Medicine (1988)
Stress Management Techniques (1988)
Overcoming Stress (1988)
Know Yourself (1988)
The Health Scandal (1988)
The 20 Minute Health Check (1989)
Sex for Everyone (1989)
Mind Over Body (1989)
Eat Green Lose Weight (1990)
Toxic Stress (1991)
Why Animal Experiments Must Stop
   (1991)
The Drugs Myth (1992)
Arthritis (1993)
Backache (1993)
Stress and Relaxation (1993)
Complete Guide to Good Sex (1993)
Why Doctors Do More Harm Than Good
   (1993)
Betrayal of Trust (1994)

Know Your Drugs (1994)
Food for Thought (1994)

Novels
The Village Cricket Tour (1990)
The Bilbury Chronicles (1992)
Bilbury Grange (1993)
Mrs Caldicot's Cabbage War (1993)
The Man Who Inherited a Golf Club
   (1993)
The Bilbury Revels (1994)
Deadline (1994)

Writing as Edward Vernon
Practice Makes Perfect (novel, 1977)
Practise What You Preach (novel, 1978)
Getting into Practice (novel, 1979)
Aphrodisiacs—An Owner's Manual (1983)
The Complete Guide to Life (1984)

As Marc Charbonnier
Tunnel (novel, 1980)

With Dr Alan C. Turin
No More Headaches (1981)

With Alice
Alice's Diary (1989)
Alice's Adventures (1992)

The traditional home doctor

Vernon Coleman

EUROPEAN
MEDICAL
JOURNAL

Dedicated to
Gill Redfearn

First published in the United Kingdom by the European Medical Journal,
Publishing House, Trinity Place, Barnstaple, Devon EX32 9HJ, England

Reprinted 1996, 1998, 1999

ISBN   0 9521492 7 3

Printed and bound in Great Britain by J. W. Arrowsmith Ltd, Bristol

Preface

When I was a small boy everyone I knew had a 'Home Doctor' on their bookshelf. Even if they only had half a dozen books the 'Home Doctor' would be there—packed with friendly, easy to use advice and full of invaluable health tips. I've always wanted to write such a book so that I could collect together all the nuggets of health care information I've acquired over the years.

During the two decades that I've been writing on health matters readers have sent me countless thousands of tips. I've accumulated thousands more by studying medical journals. And, of course, I found out quite a few for myself during the ten years that I practised as a family doctor! The tips in this book are timeless so the information it contains isn't going to go out of date. There are no fancy diagrams in this book and you won't find out how to perform a heart transplant operation either. But you will, I hope, find this book enormously useful whenever you are faced with a family health problem.

I hope that in a few years time, when it's beginning to look dog eared and well thumbed, you'll think of my *Traditional Home Doctor* as a family friend.

Vernon Coleman
January 1994
Devon, England

NOTE

This book is not intended to be, and cannot be, an alternative to personal, professional medical advice. Readers should immediately consult a trained and properly qualified health professional, whom they trust and respect, for advice about any symptom or health problem which requires diagnosis, treatment or any kind of medical attention.

While the advice and information in this book are believed to be accurate and true at the time of going to press, neither the author nor the publisher can accept any legal responsibility or liability for errors or omissions which may be made.

The traditional home doctor

ACNE

Acne runs in families and mainly affects teenagers (9 out of 10 suffer from it). Hormone changes at puberty make the skin oily and spots develop when hair follicles are blocked with oil. If bacteria are trapped under the skin red spots develop with the face, shoulders, neck and upper back most commonly involved.

Washing twice a day with a rough cloth will help keep pores clean and sunshine and artificial sun lamps may also help improve the skin. When spots become infected antibiotics are usually prescribed—often for several weeks or months at a time.

ALCOHOLISM

The liver isn't the only organ which can be damaged by too much drinking. Stomach ulcers, muscle wastage, cancer and brain disease all occur in alcoholics. Early physical symptoms of alcoholism include hand tremor, indigestion, poor appetite, impotence, fits, blackouts, memory lapses and frequent accidents. Anxiety, depression and restlessness at night are also common. Most alcoholics do enormous damage to those around them as they lie, steal and break the law. Half of road deaths are caused by people influenced by alcohol. Alcoholism is an addiction but it can be treated.

You should check that your consumption of alcohol remains within safe limits. For men the weekly limit is 21 units spread throughout the week. For women the weekly limit is 14 units spread throughout the week.

How much alcohol is there in your drink?

1 pint of ordinary strength beer or lager contains 2 units
1 pint export beer or lager contains 2.5 units
1 pint strong beer or lager contains 4 units
1 pint extra strong beer or lager contains 5 units
1 pint cider contains 3 units
1 pint strong cider contains 4 units
1 average glass of wine contains 1 unit (pub measure)

1 average glass of sherry, port or vermouth contains 1 unit (pub measure)
1 average glass of liqueur contains 1 unit (pub measure)
1 single of spirits contains 1 unit (pub measure)

ALCOHOL AND PILLS

Every week many people put their lives at risk by drinking alcohol while taking prescribed drugs.

Doctors have become sloppy and careless about providing warnings but there is no doubt that mixing booze with drugs as varied as antibiotics and tranquillisers, sleeping pills and blood pressure tablets can be lethal.

Alcohol is a powerful drug in its own right. When taken with other powerful drugs the combination can kill.

Here's what can happen if you drink alcohol while taking any of the following medicines:

High blood pressure pills

Mixing alcohol with blood pressure tablets can alter the drug's effect—with the result that your blood pressure goes out of control.

If your blood pressure goes down you could become faint and dizzy. If it goes up too much you could have a stroke.

Anti-histamines for allergies

If you drink alcohol while taking an anti-histamine the chances of you suddenly becoming drowsy are increased. Driving a car after taking an anti-histamine alone is dangerous. Driving after taking an anti-histamine and alcohol is like playing Russian roulette.

Antibiotics and anti-infectives

Some antibiotics simply fail to work as effectively if taken with alcohol. But the combination could lead to nausea, vomiting, headaches and convulsions.

Painkillers

Mixing alcohol and a painkiller could kill you.

Tranquillisers

If you drink alcohol while taking a tranquilliser your ability to think clearly and act quickly will be badly damaged. You'll be likely to make mistakes at work and be far more likely to have an accident at home or on the roads. And you'll probably feel constantly sleepy too.

Sleeping tablets

When taken with alcohol sleeping tablets can lead to coma, respiratory arrest and death.

Diuretics

Taking alcohol with a diuretic (a tablet designed to increase excretion of fluids) can lead to lowered blood pressure, dizziness and collapse.

Antidepressant

Mixing alcohol with antidepressants could produce a wide variety of symptoms. The mixture could prove deadly.

Diabetic drugs

Taking a drug for the treatment of diabetes and then drinking alcohol could lead to the diabetes going out of control—possibly fatally.

Remember, this list isn't comprehensive. Whenever you are given a prescription drug you should only drink alcohol if your doctor has given you the all clear.

If you are in any doubt *don't* drink booze while taking a medicine. It could kill you.

ALLERGIES

10 substances most likely to cause an allergy reaction and 5 common types of allergy

Allergies affect a third of the population and the problem is getting bigger every year. The number of people visiting their doctor for treatment for allergy related problems such as asthma and hay fever has doubled in recent years. Many experts believe that the incidence of allergies is going up as our environment becomes more and more polluted.

The human body has a sophisticated series of internal defence mechanisms designed to help provide protection against a vast variety of different threats. It is the immunological system which enables the human body to protect itself against infections.

Efficient as it is, however, this system will sometimes over-react to foreign substances; switching on special defences which aren't needed and producing uncomfortable and sometimes violent symptoms which are in practice more of a threat than the cause of the response!

Allergy reactions can develop to foreign substances which enter the body through the nose or the mouth or which simply come into contact with the skin. A whole range of different substances can cause allergy reactions. It is probably true to say that there is no substance in the world to which some individual has not at some time developed an allergy reaction. Pollens, dust, foods and animals are perhaps the commonest causes of reactions.

Ten substances most likely to cause an allergy reaction

1   House dust mites (found in any home, however clean).
2   Cows' milk (and dairy products such as butter, cheese and yoghurt)
3   Pollen
4   Cat and dog hair
5   Mould spores
6   Feathers and wool
7   Drugs such as penicillin
8   Perfumes of various kinds
9   Tobacco
10 Metals such as nickel (used in bra straps and jewellery)

This list isn't complete of course. Any food (eggs and wheat among them) can cause an allergy. As can any drug.

The type of allergy reaction you have depends on a number of factors. And things are complicated by the fact that anyone can suffer from one, two or even more different allergies—often producing symptoms at the same time.

Here are some of the commonest types of allergy reactions.

1   Eczema commonly occurs because of an allergy reaction which develops in the skin. Eczema in children seems to be associated with foodstuffs and experimenting with an exclusion diet can help.

2   Asthma is one of the most serious allergy diseases as it can lead to great physical distress—and can even kill. Asthma is usually caused by an allergy to pollen, dust or animals.

3   Allergic rhinitis is one of the commonest forms of allergy reactions. Someone who appears to suffer permanently from colds may well suffer from allergic rhinitis.

4   Hay fever occurs when the sufferer is allergic to something which occurs seasonally.

5   Migraine may also be caused by an allergic reaction to various foods such as chocolate, red wine or bananas. It can also be caused by tobacco. (*See also* Migraine.)

There is no doubt that some allergic reactions are easy to spot. If a child complains of itchy eyes and sneezing during the pollen season then it isn't to difficult to diagnose hay fever. If a nasty rash develops after using a brand of soap that hasn't been used before, an allergic reaction may well be the cause of the problem.

Food allergies are often easy to diagnose. For example, during the summer months strawberries are a common cause of rashes—producing a red, blotchy and itchy skin rash.

The symptoms produced by an allergy may not always be so obvious. For example, a patient with a food allergy may complain of symptoms which initially appear unconnected to the food. Vomiting, diarrhoea and stomach pains are all disorders which can occur as a result of a food allergy.

ALZHEIMER'S DISEASE

Ten things you should try to remember about Alzheimer's disease

1   Alzheimer's disease is the commonest cause of dementia or senility among people aged 65 or older. It affects one in three over 85. But Alzheimer's disease also affects men and women in their forties and fifties.

2   No one knows what causes it. There are various theories. Some claim that Alzheimer's disease is caused by aluminium poisoning. Others say that it can be caused by an infection. There is some evidence that the disease can be inherited.

3   The disease causes nerve cells in the brain to stop working properly—and also makes the brain shrink.

4   The first symptom is usually forgetfulness. Sufferers often try to jog their memories by writing lists. The loss of memory is so bad that it makes many Alzheimer's patients feel anxious and depressed. Memory for long ago events is not so badly affected as memory for recent events: sufferers can remember what happened fifty years ago but can't remember something that happened yesterday.

5   Next, sufferers become disorientated. They don't know where they are and may lose their way even in their own homes. They have difficulty in finding the right word when speaking or writing and their ability to do simple sums declines.

6   In the final stage Alzheimer's sufferers become very confused. They may become paranoid and may have hallucinations. Incontinence is also a common problem. At this stage victims often need full time nursing care.

7   Simple tests are often done to measure mental agility. Here's one that psychiatrists often use: Start with 100 and subtract 7 from it. That gives you 93. In the early stages of Alzheimer's disease patients will have difficulty in remembering the name of the Prime Minister. In the later stages

they'll have difficulty in remembering their own name.

8 Brain scans are sometimes done to confirm the diagnosis. A patient suffering from Alzheimer's disease will usually have a brain which has shrunk in size.

9 There is no effective treatment though patients are encouraged to be as active as possible. Eating well and exercising often are important, as are trying to maintain interests and hobbies.

10 Victims tend to live a long time and relatives suffer enormously as they struggle to look after someone they love whose personality may well be unrecognisable.

ANAEMIA

If the amount of oxygen carrying pigment—haemoglobin—in your blood falls too low then you will be anaemic. Haemoglobin carries oxygen into your body and without it you will feel tired and breathless and look pale. There are many possible causes but regular bleeding (e.g. heavy monthly periods in women) or a diet that lacks iron are two of the commonest. Foods which are rich in iron, such as wholemeal bread, beans, green vegetables and fruit, help prevent—and treat—diet induced iron deficiency anaemia.

ANOREXIA NERVOSA

7 tell tale symptoms

Anorexia nervosa is a reluctance to eat—and a consequent severe weight loss which is often blamed on slimming but usually thought to be caused by psychological problems. Patients are often hard working, obsessional and desperate to succeed. Symptoms (apart from severe weight loss) include weakness, dry skin and fine hair on the body. Anorexia nervosa needs to be treated very seriously because it can kill—1 in 20 sufferers die or commit suicide.

The tell tale symptoms of anorexia nervosa are:

1   a dramatic weight loss: sufferers often lose a quarter of their weight

2   an obsession with dieting: however thin they get, anorexia nervosa sufferers still claim that they need to lose weight

3   overactivity: sufferers often fidget a lot and have difficulty in getting to sleep at night

4   an obsession with food: surprisingly, many anorexia nervosa patients spend hours preparing food for other people

5   girls who suffer from anorexia nervosa stop menstruating

6   head hair often disappears but a fine, downy hair may appear on the patient's body

7   sufferers often complain of feeling cold—even though everyone else thinks it's warm

The victims of anorexia nervosa are usually teenage girls (although boys can get it) and the average age is around 17. The disorder is so common that there is likely to be at least one sufferer in every large school.

Just what causes anorexia nervosa is uncertain. Some experts say that the disease affects girls who are frightened of growing up and who lack confidence in themselves. Some say that girls who push themselves too hard and have high expectations are most likely to suffer. Others say that an obsession with losing weight can lead to anorexia nervosa.

One of the few things we know for certain is that anorexia nervosa is common among girls who want to become models, actresses or dancers.

Whatever the cause may be, anorexia nervosa can be a dangerous disease. If a girl with the disease doesn't get treated she may literally starve herself to death. So, getting help is vital. Don't listen to people who say that you can cure this disease by taking special supplements. This is a disorder which requires very skilled, very specialised help.

Anorexia nervosa can be treated. But the deep rooted fears which drive girls to anorexia nervosa are powerful. Girls who have the disease often become very cunning as they attempt to cheat the people who want to help them. Experts know that girls with anorexia nervosa will often hide food or deliberately make themselves sick if they are forced to eat; they will frequently insist that they neither need nor want help.

Arthritis

9 ways you can help yourself

Each of 200 joints in the human body can be affected by arthritis. Joints normally consist of two bones—each one capped with layer of white, smooth, gristly cartilage. The two bone ends are enclosed within a capsule and surrounded by lubricating fluid. Normally joints can repair themselves and replenish their own supplies of fluid. But joints can become diseased or worn out. There are over one hundred different types of arthritis. Symptoms usually include stiffness, swelling and pain.

Although arthritis is usually incurable the symptoms can often be controlled by a mixture of diet, gentle exercise (stopping for pain) and drugs. A vegetarian diet has been shown to help arthritics.

Many people assume that arthritis is a disease that only affects the elderly but anyone over 25 years of age has a 1 in 4 chance of being an arthritis sufferer.

Few diseases affect as many people as arthritis. Few cause as much pain, discomfort and disablement. And few are the subject of so many myths and so much misunderstanding.

Millions of people already suffer from arthritis. Many are in constant pain. Some are severely disabled. Most suffer occasional agonies.

There are over one hundred different types of arthritis. But the two commonest are rheumatoid arthritis and osteoarthritis.

Rheumatoid arthritis usually affects the smaller joints in the body—particularly the joints of the hands and wrist. A dozen or more separate joints may be affected. Pain, tenderness, swelling and stiffness are the most common symptoms. Three times as many women as men are affected and women between the ages of 25 and 50 are the main sufferers.

Osteoarthritis is an almost inevitable result of growing old. It commonly strikes between the ages of 50 and 60 and, like rheumatoid arthritis, it affects more women than men. It develops as the cartilage which normally stops bones from rubbing together is worn away. Osteoarthritis can be inherited and is made worse by overweight but it commonly develops in joints which get a lot of wear and tear, so the joints most commonly affected are the knees, hands, feet and hips.

If you go to your doctor complaining of the symptoms of arthritis he will probably prescribe a drug for you. But you should be aware that some of the products which are most widely used can cause serious side effects. And, sadly, there is still no real 'cure' for any of the arthritis diseases. Drug companies are constantly producing new 'wonder' drugs for which great things are promised. But many have had to be withdrawn after dangerous—sometimes lethal—side effects have developed.

Some experts still believe that ordinary soluble aspirin tablets are still among the best ways to control the painful symptoms of arthritis.

There are many things you can do yourself to help minimise the pain and to help control the stiffness and discomfort.

1   When the pain of your arthritis is bad then you should rest. Exercising sore or painful joints can damage them. But when the pain goes away you should exercise your joints as much as you can. Movement will help to ensure that your joints do not become too stiff.

2   If you are using drugs to help control your pain remember that you will almost certainly need to take your pills *regularly.* And check frequently with your doctor that you are taking the correct dosage. Since *all* the drugs used to treat arthritis can cause side effects, make sure that you tell your doctor about any unusual symptoms.

3   If you suffer from *any* arthritis in *any* joint try hard to lose excess weight. Every pound of unwanted fat that you carry will make your arthritis worse. Many overweight patients who are crippled by their arthritis would be able to walk if

they would make a real effort to lose weight.

4   When your joints are painful or sore try to keep them warm. Heat will relieve pain and stiffness. You can get the heat you need from a warm bath, a hot water bottle or a heat lamp. Many arthritis sufferers find that swimming— particularly in warm water—helps them enormously.

5   Exercise regularly—it will help to keep your joints in good condition. Swimming in warm water is the best form of exercise you can do. Walking is also good but do try to walk on soft ground rather than on hard roads or pavements (the shock of walking—or even worse jogging—on hard surfaces can do a considerable amount of joint damage).

6   If you suffer from a lot of pain ask your doctor to arrange for you to borrow a TENS machine from a local pain clinic (there are pain clinics at most large hospitals). In one research study doctors found that TENS machines were two and a half times as effective as paracetamol at relieving pain. (TENS machines are small battery operated devices that use electricity to interfere with pain impulses.)

7   Learn how to relax. A report published in America showed that when patients with arthritis learn how to relax properly they suffer considerably less pain. And make sure that you put plenty of fun into your life! Doctors have also shown that laughter helps to control pain—and even to cure joint damage.

8   You can strengthen your joints with specific exercises. For example, you may be able to strengthen your knees by lying flat on your back, lifting your legs into the air and pedalling an imaginary bicycle. You should always stop at the slightest hint of pain when you are exercising and never begin any exercise programme without asking your doctor about it first.

9   Some experts now believe that arthritis sufferers may benefit from following a vegetarian diet. Talk to your doctor or ask for an appointment to see a dietician if you aren't sure how to prepare a healthy, vegetarian diet. Or see my book,

Food for Thought: Your Guide to Healthy Eating (published by the European Medical Journal).

Joint replacement operations are extremely effective these days. Operations on arthritic hips are commonplace and thousands of patients who were crippled can now walk again. If your symptoms are disabling talk to your doctor about whether or not surgery would help you.

ASTHMA
including 6 tips to help you cope

Asthma is one of the most common long term illnesses but it is the subject of a great many misconceptions—and the confusion which sometimes surrounds it means that patients with asthma often suffer unnecessarily.

Asthma develops because the tubes which carry air into the lungs become obstructed. Some inborn factor means that the muscles which surround the air passages react too rapidly and too easily, while the lining inside the passageways has a tendency to swell. Triggered by external factors which I will describe later the linings swell and the muscle walls contract. The inevitable result is a narrowing of the airways.

The four basic signs and symptoms which identify the asthma sufferer are:

❖ Breathlessness—the patient usually feels as though he would like to get more air into his chest but cannot. It is a frightening feeling which should never be underestimated.

❖ Most patients with asthma will wheeze. The wheezing is most obvious when they breathe out.

❖ The majority of asthma sufferers cough a great deal.

❖ The breathlessness, the wheezing and the coughing all come and go. Occasionally, the symptoms will disappear entirely. Sometimes just one symptom will be present. On other occasions all three symptoms will occur together.

The majority of individuals who get asthma suffer from

allergic asthma. They wheeze and cough and get breathless because they have been in contact with something to which they are allergic. Grasses, pollen, house dust, cat fur, feathers, dogs, rabbits and horses are some of the most common causes.

When asthma is produced by an allergen the body reacts internally in much the same way that it can react externally. If a woman uses eye make up to which she is allergic, the tissues around her eyes will become red and swollen. Although the mechanism may be different a similar sort of thing happens in allergic asthma. The passageways inside the lungs simply react by swelling to an allergen which has been breathed in through the nose or mouth. And the swollen, irritated air passageways impede the air that is trying to get through. Hence the breathlessness and the wheezing.

If these symptoms obviously occur whenever the sufferer is in contact with a particular object or pet then it isn't too difficult to diagnose the problem. The child who wheezes everytime he sleeps on feather pillows is pretty clearly allergic to feathers while the child who wheezes every time she strokes Grandma's cat is obviously allergic to Grandma's cat. (Unfortunately, it isn't always this easy to find a link between the asthma and the cause).

There are many other possible causes of asthma in addition to allergy. Infections, for example, can make wheezing and breathlessness much worse. The existence of a link between chest infections and asthma means that any asthmatic child who gets a cold should, perhaps, be treated with a little extra care.

If mild chest infections regularly seem to lead to attacks of asthma, it is probably a good idea to treat those infections with antibiotics.

The quality of air individuals breathe can also have a dramatic effect on their susceptibility to asthma. It is well known that very cold air, dry air or polluted air (for example, polluted by cigarette smoke) can produce asthma or make asthma worse.

It is perhaps less well known that air heated by gas or polluted by cooking smells, road works, factories or heavy traffic can also produce or exacerbate an asthma attack.

Finally, it is extremely important to remember that asthma can quite definitely be made worse by emotional upsets, by stress and by worry of all kinds. Anyone who wheezes or who gets breathless a good deal of the time and for no very obvious reason may well be suffering from anxiety induced asthma. Parents and teachers will often put children under too much pressure to do well. When they do, asthma is often the result. It is important to remember, by the way, that children are very aware of moods. If there is a lot of tension in the home, a child who is at all susceptible to asthma may well begin to wheeze and cough.

Asthma can be inherited. Doctors who have studied the statistics claim that if one or both parents suffered from asthma when they were children, or suffer from asthma now, then a child has a one in ten chance of suffering too. Oddly, it doesn't seem to make any difference to a child's chances of getting asthma whether one or both parents were sufferers. Asthma is not infectious, by the way.

If there is no family history of asthma then about one in twenty children are affected. Boys seem slightly more likely to suffer than girls and if a child is going to suffer then he will probably have had his first symptoms by the time he has reached the age of five years.

There is, however, some good news.

Three out of four childhood sufferers of asthma will grow out of their asthma. Put that another way: if you have a child with asthma he has only a 25% chance of continuing to suffer from it when he grows up.

If you have a child with asthma then sooner or later someone will probably tell you that he is bound to get eczema too. It is true that there is a link between the two diseases. Both can be produced by allergy reactions and so a child who suffers from one may well suffer from the other.

Despite this link it is not true to say that all children with asthma will automatically get eczema. (Nor is it true that all children with eczema will get asthma). When the two diseases do go together it is usually the eczema that comes first.

6 tips to help conquer asthma

1   By and large you should ignore all the good advice and the warnings you are given by well meaning friends and relatives. If you find yourself suffocating under a blanket of unwanted advice just tell your friends that the real problem is 'recurrent paroxysmal dyspnoea' (that is medical jargon for repeated attacks of breathlessness—and it should give you a breather).

2   If you can find out what is causing the symptoms then you will have taken a major step forward. Your doctor may be able to refer you to a clinic where they can do special tests. Meanwhile, to reduce the risks use cotton or nylon bedlinen rather than woollen, avoid feather pillows and be careful to clear away all the dust from the tops of wardrobes etc. Keep doors shut when you are cooking (so that the fumes don't spread around the house) and don't let people smoke in your house.

3   The question of what to do about pets is a difficult one. If you know that you are allergic to a specific pet then you have to decide what to do: to put up with the suffering or to find the pet another home. In general, if you have a child with asthma it is probably best not to buy any pets.

4   Asthmatic children should be encouraged to take an active part in games and exercise programmes.

5   There is a strong temptation to over protect the asthmatic child. Try and resist it. Over protected children tend to suffer more because they become conscious that their parents are worrying and so they start worrying. Worry always exacerbates asthma.

6   If you are wheezing and can't stop wheezing, you must call your doctor. Learn to get the best out of your doctor. There are many useful prescription drugs available—but make sure that these are used as sparingly as possible. Prescribable drugs for asthma fall into two categories: those intended to relieve symptoms and those intended to prevent symptoms developing. Make sure that you know whether a prescribed drug

needs to be given continuously or only in case of problems. Remember that attacks of asthma often seem to start at night, at weekends or when you are away on holiday. This is not just a cruel coincidence—it is a consequence of the fact that stress is often higher at these times. You will save yourself much worry if you keep a small stock with you of whatever drugs your doctor considers appropriate. You can measure the effectiveness of treatment yourself by using a special meter at home.

BABY DEVELOPMENT

Baby's first eighteen months: your quick guide to how your baby should develop

All children develop at different rates and there is really no such thing as a 'normal' rate of development. Some geniuses started out in life rather slowly!

However, there are some fairly well established stages of development and you should see your doctor for reassurance if your child hasn't reached the appropriate milestones at the ages listed below.

By the time he's 6 months old your baby should be able to:
- roll over by himself
- stand on his own legs if you support him and hold his hands or arms
- sit up (with a little help)
- hold up his head and look around
- stare at things and follow people with his eyes
- reach out for toys with one or both hands
- put things in his mouth
- move things from one hand to the other
- shake, bang and rattle (and destroy) things he's picked up
- look at himself in a mirror
- play (and enjoy) simple games such as peek–a–boo
- turn his head in the direction of a noise
- laugh, gurgle and make a variety of noises

- recognise when his mother is pleased or cross with him

By the time he is 9 months old your baby should be able to:
- sit without support
- try to crawl around
- pull himself up to a standing position
- walk if supported
- hold tightly onto objects (sometimes having difficulty in letting go)
- hunt for toys that are hidden
- wave goodbye
- clap his hands together
- appreciate what 'no' means (though he won't necessarily obey)
- make sounds such as mama and dada which are comprehensible only to a select circle of adults
- make specific noises when he wants something
- try to feed himself

By the time he is 12 months old your baby should be able to:
- crawl around on his hands and knees
- walk (possibly rather hesitantly and uncertainly)
- bang two objects together (and enjoy the noise)
- pick up and put down small objects quite easily
- throw things (though probably not accurately)
- demonstrate affection to people he knows and likes
- play simple games
- respond when he hears his own name
- say two or three words
- talk cheerily to himself
- know what common household objects are used for

By the time he is 18 months old your baby should be able to:
- walk quite well, maybe even run
- walk upstairs with one hand held
- stoop to pick things up
- crawl backwards downstairs
- turn the pages of a book

- scribble with crayons
- build a tower of three building blocks
- say between 6 and 20 words
- occasionally understand things that are said to him
- explore his surroundings
- look at a picture book
- put things into boxes (and take them out again)
- take off his shoes and socks
- use a spoon
- use a cup
- have a tantrum and exhibit the first signs of bad temper

Teeth

The first teeth usually appear at the age of about six months. The incisors at the front of the mouth invariably appear first, with the incisors in the lower jaw usually appearing before those in the upper jaw. By the age of one there are usually teeth on each side of the incisors, in both the lower and upper jaws. The first molars, the large teeth at the back of the jaws, appear in the first few months of a child's second year of life. The canines fill in the gap between the incisors and the first molars by the time a child is about eighteen months old. The second molars come about or just after the age of two. Those first milk teeth will usually last a child until 6 or 8 years of age. Then the permanent teeth will start to appear.

BABY EMERGENCY

How to cope if you find that your baby has stopped breathing

Many babies could be saved if parents knew how to perform simple resuscitation techniques. There isn't time to wait for a doctor or ambulance driver to arrive when a baby stops breathing. Follow the proper resuscitation procedure and you could save your baby's life in an emergency.

This technique is designed for babies or children under the age of two years.

1 Check if your baby is breathing by picking him up, calling to him or touching the soles of his feet. If there is no response start to resuscitate straight away.

2 Put your baby on a firm surface.

3 Carefully clear any obstruction from his nose and mouth. Do not touch the back of his throat.

4 Support the back of your baby's neck with one hand and use the other hand to tilt his head backwards slightly.

5 Seal your lips around your baby's mouth and nose and puff gently into his lungs twenty times a minute. His chest should rise as you breathe into his body. Remove your mouth after each puff of breath to allow him to breathe out.

6 If your baby's heart has stopped beating press down just below the centre of his breastbone (just below the mid-point of an imaginary line joining his two nipples)—using two fingers. You should push down for half an inch to an inch. You need to do this five times for every puff of breath you blow into your baby's lungs.

BABY FEEDING

20 facts every woman should know to help her choose between breast or bottle feeding

1 Breast size has nothing to do with milk production. Women with small breasts can feed their babies very successfully. Very large breasts often contain a great deal of fat—which has nothing to do with milk production.

2 Human milk is quite different from other types of milk. It contains a unique mixture of water, protein, fat, lactose, minerals and vitamins. It is specially designed for babies.

3 The breast milk a mum produces immediately after her baby is born is rich in antibodies which protect a newborn baby against infection.

4 By and large the more milk a baby takes the more milk your breasts will produce.

5   Breast fed babies are less likely to develop eczema than bottle fed babies (8% of breast fed babies get eczema compared to 50% of bottle fed babies).

6   Babies fed on breast milk are less likely to develop intestinal infections.

7   Breast feeding reduces the chances of your getting pregnant—but it isn't a reliable contraceptive.

8   Breast fed babies are less likely to get fat in later life.

9   If your baby doesn't take all the milk you produce the excess can be gently squeezed out and, if you like, fed to your baby on a spoon or in a cup.

10 Breast feeding will probably increase the size of your bust. Your breasts and your nipples may remain larger when you have finished feeding.

11 To stop one breast swelling it is important to make sure that your baby feeds at each breast in turn—ten minutes at each breast is usually just about right.

12 If the milk production stops, continued sucking by your baby should start the milk flow again.

13 If you are breast feeding you shouldn't drink alcohol or take pills (unless your doctor says it is definitely all right) since the alcohol or drugs may appear in your milk. You may need to increase your calorie intake by up to 40% if you are breast feeding.

14 The incidence of breast cancer is lower among women who have breast fed.

15 Women who breast feed usually notice that their stomachs get flatter again more quickly after the pregnancy.

16 Babies fed on breast milk usually soil their nappies less than bottle fed babies.

17 If milk ducts get blocked a hard, painful area can develop within the breast.

18 If you feed your baby by bottle hold him close while you do so—this way you won't deny your baby the bonding that takes place during breast feeding.

19 If preparing bottle feeds always follow the manufacturer's instructions carefully. Adding extra milk powder—or sugar—will harm your baby.

20 One big advantage with bottle feeding is that anyone can do it—it doesn't have to be mum. You can leave bottles prepared in the fridge. And *he* can get up at night to feed the baby.

☞ *See also* Weaning; Wind

BABY NOTES

25 things you should know about a newborn baby

1 All newborn babies have a pug nose. The bridge of the nose isn't there at birth—it grows later—so babies have a small 'button' nose.

2 Nearly all babies are born with blue or blue–gray eyes. Permanent eye colouration develops during the following months.

3 Babies may cry a lot but they don't produce any tears. There is moisture to lubricate and clean the eyes but proper tears don't start to appear until the baby is between three and twelve weeks of age.

4 Any hair that is on your newborn baby's head will soon fall out—to be replaced by permanent hair (which may be of an entirely different colour) at about six months.

5 All newborn babies—even black ones—have a ruddy complexion. This is because their blood contains a high number of red blood cells.

6 Four out of ten babies are born with at least one birthmark.

7 The commonest day of the week for babies to be born is Tuesday. Fewer babies are born on Saturday or Sunday than on any other day of the week (though this may simply be because doctors and midwives don't like working weekends).

8   Babies have a strongly developed sense of smell. By the time he is one week old a baby can identify his mother by her smell.

9   Newborn babies are genetically programmed to respond to the human voice—especially female voices. Babies learn to distinguish between different sounds very quickly.

10   Few babies have much of a sense of taste—though most prefer sweet tasting liquids.

11   Babies have very poor eyesight. Their eyes are focused on a spot about eight inches away—so you need to get really close if your baby is to see you clearly. Babies prefer looking at curved lines rather than straight lines.

12   Contrary to the old wives' tale, babies are not colour blind. They prefer strong primary colours—particularly red and blue.

13   The heart of a newborn baby beats between 130 and 160 times a minute (about twice that of a normal adult).

14   Babies breathe much faster than adults—30 to 50 times a minute compared to an adult's 15 to 20 times a minute.

15   Babies often sneeze and snort in their sleep to clear their nasal passages. Only later on can babies breathe through their mouth if their nose is blocked. To minimise the problem keep the air in the home as clear and as smoke and dust free as possible.

16   Although babies get some immunity—and protection from infection—from their mothers, they are still very vulnerable to colds. Keep anyone with a cold away from your baby.

17   Babies have very small stomachs. An 8lb baby can get 3 ounces of milk into its stomach. It is the small size of the stomach that explains why 95% of all babies occasionally vomit everything they have eaten. So babies need small feeds regularly (every three or four hours) rather than large feeds occasionally.

18   Nearly every newborn baby gets wind—and colic—that lasts for the first three months of its life.

19 Newborn babies spend between 15 and 20 hours a day sleeping—in bouts of sleep lasting 20 minutes to 5 hours.

20 In the first year of his life your baby will triple his weight, increase his length by 50%, double the size of his brain and create every nerve cell he will ever have.

21 Babies respond well to touch—which stimulates the production of growth promoting hormones and helps the body become more responsive to these hormones. In one survey it was shown that premature babies who were touched regularly showed 47% more weight gain.

22 Babies are often nervous—even fearful—of new foods. To enable your baby to overcome his fears allow him to play with the food a little before eating it. You may be able to encourage a baby to try a new food by putting a small amount of food on his index finger and then gently guiding his index finger into his mouth.

23 If a baby suddenly starts to refuse a once favourite food it probably means that he is bored with it and would appreciate a little variation in his diet.

24 Teething can start when your baby is just three months old.

25 Babies sometimes need background noise to help them get to sleep (the womb is not the quietest place in the world). Some sounds that are known to relax and soothe babies include: a recording of their mother's heartbeat; the sound of a clock ticking; a recording of a stream, waterfall or sea; a vacuum cleaner; air bubbling through a fish tank; running water from a tap.

BABY WARNING SIGNS

Symptoms that mean you should call the doctor

Every parent who has a baby worries when it cries, doesn't take a feed properly or seems off colour. 'Is it serious?' and 'Do I need to call the doctor?' are the two questions every mum asks herself.

Parents are often slow to ask for medical advice from their doctor when their baby is ill. Some are frightened to telephone for advice because they don't like to bother the doctor. Others worry about facing the receptionist. Many simply don't know what to look for.

If your baby or young child has any of the following symptoms then you should consult your doctor straight away. This list is not exhaustive, of course. But it does contain some of the most important warning signs.

- unexplained crying or screaming, particularly crying that is persistent or unusual; you should also call for help if your baby's cry seems in any way unusual

- lying still and losing his usual interest in the world

- drowsiness—you must get advice if your baby doesn't seem as alert or as awake as usual

- blood on your baby's nappy or around his bottom

- wheezing (a whistling noise that occurs when your baby breaths out) or breathing difficulties or abnormalities mean that you should call your doctor

- high temperature

- fits or convulsions

- flushing or pallor; you should talk to your doctor if your baby's colour is unusual

- going off his or her food

- vomiting; in particular you should get help if your baby has vomited after two or more feeds or if the vomit looks a green colour (vomit that looks green possibly contains bile and suggests that there could possibly be an obstruction of some kind)

- diarrhoea

- if, when you pick your baby up, he seems floppy or seems to be having more difficulty than usual in holding his head up, ring for help

- any sign of neck stiffness means that you should call your doctor straight away

- you should get help if your baby isn't drinking properly or is passing less urine than usual
- if your baby is behaving unusually, taking less interest than usual in his surroundings or failing to respond in his normal way, you should get advice straight away
- failing to develop properly

Remember that problems that affect babies can develop rapidly. Do not be tempted to wait 24 hours to 'see what happens'.

I believe that if more parents called for medical help sooner rather than later, a number of disasters could be prevented.

You should even call your doctor for help if you only think that something is wrong—even if you can't quite put your finger on what it is. Mothers, in particular, know their babies better than anyone else. Their instincts are too often right to be ignored.

(*Note:* Do remember that sometimes perfectly healthy babies will show one or more of the signs I have listed above. There isn't necessarily anything for you to worry about—but getting help is essential.)

BACKACHE

7 ways to avoid it & 8 ways to conquer it

At least eight out of ten cases of backache are caused by muscle tension—usually produced by poor posture, stress or carelessness. And so in eight out of ten cases backache can be avoided. Here's how!

1 *Be careful how you sit*

   Sit with your back straight and never stay in the same position for more than an hour—get up, stretch and walk about.

2 *Be careful how you stand*

   Don't stand for long periods: change your position occasionally.

3 *Be careful in bed*

A firm mattress will keep your back in good condition. If your mattress is soggy put a board under it to make it firmer.

4 *Be careful when working or lifting*

Lift or pick things up bending at the knees, not at the waist—keep your back straight.

☞ *Ten tips for lifting without damaging your back*

Lifting—or trying to lift—heavy objects is a major cause of back trouble. Follow these tips to help protect your back.

1   There is no acceptable definition of heavy. Any load can damage your back if you lift in the wrong way. Always lift carefully and always think before lifting.

2   Whenever possible work out a way to minimise the effort required. If there is a mechanical hoist available—use it. If you can use a trolley or barrow then use one. Unload cupboards and take heavy furniture apart whenever possible. If there is nothing on the object to hold onto then use a sling or put a strong rope underneath it. If there is help available then wait until it arrives. Plan to lift and move heavy objects in gentle, easy stages. Stop if you feel tired— that is when accidents happen.

3   If you have to move a heavy weight on a trolley remember that pulling usually puts less strain on your body than pushing.

4   Make sure that you wear shoes with non slip soles. Do not try lifting or carrying heavy weights while wearing high heels. If possible wear shoes that provide proper protection in case something heavy drops on your feet. And make sure that you use gloves that provide a good grip. Don't try lifting in unusually loose or unusually tight clothing, in clothing that restricts your movements in any way or in clothing that might 'catch' on a protrusion.

5   Stand close to the object you want to lift with your feet apart to improve your balance. Put one foot slightly ahead of the other.

6   Bend your hips and your knees and keep your back straight

and your shoulders level and in line with your pelvis. Pick up the object you are lifting with the whole of your hand (rather than just your finger tips) and keep your arms close in to your body. A weight held out at arms' length puts ten times the strain on your spine as a weight held close to your body.

7 Brace your abdominal muscles and then lift the object by straightening your knees. If you are trying to lift something very heavy halve the stress by lifting one end first. If you have to turn move your feet as well as your body and make sure that you do not twist or bend your body while lifting.

8 Try to lift smoothly. And remember to keep the object close to your body all the time that you are holding it.

9 If the object is too heavy for you put it down straight away.

10 When putting a load down lower yourself by bending your knees and squatting. Do not bend your back when putting something down—this is when injuries often happen.

5 *Exercise regularly*

Swimming and walking will help build up your back muscles and keep your ligaments in good condition

6 *Diet if you are overweight*

Ten pounds of excess weight on your abdomen is equivalent to a pressure of 100 pounds of additional weight inside your spine.

7 *Avoid high heels*

Women who wear high heels all the time can put their spines out of line and give themselves long term back problems.

And now here are some ways to combat backache.

Eight ways to conquer backache

1 Ask your doctor for help immediately.

2 Rest is vital. And you must lie flat and rest in bed if you are in pain. Research has shown that back sufferers who get up

too soon suffer from relapses.

3   Take painkillers. Aspirin is one of the best and most effective remedies for backache. Soluble aspirin tablets are less
likely to cause side effects than solid tablets. Do take the
recommended dosage.

4   Use heat. Few things soothe muscular backache as effectively as lying in a bath full of warm water. Alternatively
heat your bed with an electric blanket (though not while
you're in it). Or apply heat directly to the painful area by
using heated towels, a sun lamp or an old fashioned hot
water bottle.

5   Try ice. According to a specialist at the Boston Pain Clinic
in America 78% of back pain sufferers get significant pain
relief—for up to four hours—by massaging with ice. Put
crushed ice into a hot water bottle or wrap ice cubes in a
towel. Then rub the ice over the affected area. But don't
keep the ice in contact with your skin for long or it will
burn!

6   Buy a rocking chair. According to a specialist at the Royal
College of Surgeons a rocking chair stimulates the production of nerve impulses which provide effective and
continuous relief for back pain sufferers.

7   Learn to relax. Many cases of backache are caused by stress
and pressure. Spend some time learning how to relax—and
avoiding unnecessary stress—and you may be able to avoid
the muscle tensions that lead to back pain.

8   Buy or borrow a TENS machine. TENS machines
(Transcutaneous Electrical Nerve Stimulators) send out
nerve impulses which block pain messages. Research has
shown that up to 95% of patients get pain relief with these
gadgets which run off small batteries and seem free of side
effects. They're still not widely available (drug companies
don't like them because they threaten their profits) but you
should be able to borrow one by getting your doctor to
refer you to your nearest hospital pain clinic.

BAD BREATH

4 tips to help overcome it

Catarrh, sinusitis, infected gums, dirty teeth, indigestion and constipation are some of the commonest causes of bad breath (also known as halitosis). The treatment depends upon the cause.

1   Good dental care is probably the simplest way to deal with the majority of cases of bad breath. Make sure that you clean your teeth properly and regularly. Visit your dentist for a check up.

2   If your dentist can't find a cause—or a solution—then ask your doctor for help.

3   As a temporary solution you can make a useful mouthwash by putting half a teaspoonful of salt into a glass of warm water. To make the mouthwash a little more palatable simply add a drop of peppermint oil to the glass of water.

4   Chewing a sprig of parsley will also provide temporary help.

BALDNESS

See Hair problems

BIRTHMARKS

Birthmarks are the result of slight flaws in the development process and there are many different types. Some birthmarks result from flaws in the development of blood vessels while others are the result of flaws in the distribution of skin pigments. The only thing that these skin lesions have in common is that they are all visible. (Not all birthmarks are present at birth for the type of mark known as cavernous haemangioma sometimes only becomes visible a week or two after the baby's birth).

The cavernous haemangioma is more widely known as the strawberry birthmark. The lesion is usually pink or bright red and it is clearly raised above the level of the skin so that it almost looks like the surface of a strawberry. Strawberry birthmarks can appear anywhere on the body and for the first few months of a child's life they continue to grow in size. They look very dramatic and can be most worrying for parents who haven't seen anything like them before. By the time a child reaches the age of ten most strawberry birthmarks will have disappeared completely. There is not usually any need for either surgical or medical treatment. About ten per cent of all babies seem to have strawberry birthmarks.

Another common lesion that usually disappears by itself is the blue grey discoloration which looks rather like a bruise. Known as Mongolian spots, these lesions are commonest at the base of the spine. They are found most frequently on babies with darker skins. These marks usually disappear by the time a child reaches the age of four.

The marks known as naevus simplex (also known as salmon patches, angels' kisses or stork bites) are light red areas which also tend to disappear spontaneously—usually within twelve months or so.

The commonest type of birthmarks that don't disappear themselves are the capillary haemangiomas. Known as port wine stains because they are flat, purple and do, indeed, look as though they have been made by the spilling of a rich, red wine they occur most commonly on the face—usually affecting one side only.

Port wine stains can be quite worrying but one really effective remedy is to use a waterproof cosmetic camouflage cream. A specialist beautician or a dermatologist is usually able to explain how best to mix different colours so as to produce a cream which most effectively matches the colour of the patient's own skin.

BITES AND STINGS

Bees, wasps, jellyfish and nettles sting. Animals, snakes, mosquitos, gnats, fleas, lice and ticks bite.

1 BEE STINGS

The unique fact about bee stings is that when the bee has sunk its stinger into the skin it cannot withdraw it again. It disembowels itself leaving behind the barb and the venom sac. The sac continues to discharge venom into the victim long after the bee has flown away. Since drop for drop the venom of the bee is said to be just as potent as that of the rattlesnake it is obviously important to try and get the sac out of the skin as soon as possible.

It's best not to do this by pulling the barb straight out of the skin since there is a good chance that you'll only squeeze the remaining venom into the skin. It is much safer to try and tease the stinger out sideways using a sterilised needle or a pair of tweezers. If you can't see what you're doing then use a magnifying glass.

Once the stinger and the venom sac have been removed there isn't a lot more you can do. A cold dressing, a dab of calamine lotion or a piece of ice will do as much good as anything else.

2 WASP STINGS

Unlike the bee the wasp retains its barb after an attack and can sting again. There is no specific treatment for a single wasp—I suggest that you treat a wasp sting as recommended above for bee stings. I don't recommend antihistamine creams as they can produce allergic reactions of their own.

3 NETTLE STINGS

These are uncomfortable but rarely serious. If you can't get hold of calamine lotion or a cold dressing you can try the old remedy of rubbing the area with a dock leaf.

4 ANIMAL BITES

The area of the wound should be cleaned as soon as possible—either with running water or with a liquid antiseptic. Because of the risk of tetanus it is important that anyone who is unprotected should have a vaccination jab. Animal bites are rarely serious but because of the risk of infection it is usually wise to seek medical advice. If rabies is present in your country you should always seek medical advice after a dog bite. You should identify the dog and its owner.

5 SNAKE BITES

Seek medical advice as soon as possible. Keep the victim calm and quiet and, if possible, cool the bitten area with ice or cold water. If the snake was killed during the attack then keep it for identification purposes.

6 MOSQUITOS AND GNATS

Try not to scratch the bites as this will increase the risk of infection. Minimise the irritation by using a cold dressing or calamine lotion. If you are bitten by a mosquito in an area where malaria is known then you should seek medical advice as soon as possible. You should also see a doctor if any symptoms arise within the subsequent 6 months.

There are several things which make some individuals more attractive to insects than others. Occasionally an individual who is taking a drug of some kind will excrete an especially attractive sort of smell. Sometimes a perfume may prove irresistible. But if you are always bothered more than other people by insects, it may be because of something you wear. Yellow clothing always seems to attract more insects than anything else. Do you usually wear a yellow shirt, jumper, coat or anorak? If so—try to wear something rather darker next time you go out.

7 FLEAS, LICE, TICKS AND BEDBUGS

There is no specific treatment for these bites. All you can do is soothe the inflamed area, and then try to get rid of the creatures responsible!

BLEEDING

Emergency advice on how to stop it

In an emergency, when blood is being lost at a great rate, the most effective form of first aid is the simplest: press as hard as you can on the bleeding point. If you have time to make a nice, neat pad out of a piece of freshly laundered cloth, that is fine, but if you don't have time then just press directly onto the wound. The risk of infection will be lower than the risk of the patient bleeding to death. Every ten minutes or so remove the pressure a little to allow blood into the surrounding tissues. To slow down bleeding in one particular part of the body it helps to raise the bleeding area above the rest of the body. So, for example, if a patient has a bleeding hand you can slow down blood loss by raising the hand as high as possible into the air. In any case of bleeding you should, of course, seek help as soon as possible.

BOILS, CARBUNCLES AND STYES

The body is covered with thousands of very tiny hairs, sebaceous glands which are designed to help keep the skin oily and supple, and sweat glands which have the job of helping to control the internal body temperature.

If a hair root, a sweat gland or a sebaceous gland become infected then a pimple or spot will develop. If the infection is not contained and the gland or hair follicle turns into a swollen, painful, hot, red lump then that is a boil. If there are several boils together, or if one boil has several heads, that is a carbuncle. A stye, by the way, is simply a boil that is perched on the edge of an eyelid.

It is no coincidence that boils commonly develop in painful and inconvenient sites—such as the back of the neck where the skin is rubbed by the collar. They develop in these uncomfortable places because of the constant rubbing and irritation of the skin.

If a boil develops, the first thing you must do is resist the temptation to squeeze it. Pushing and pressing on a boil is just as likely to send infected material deeper into the skin as it is to force the pus out into the open, particularly in the early stages.

You must also try to resist the temptation to smear the boil, spot or carbuncle with inches of antiseptic cream. You aren't very likely to be able to eradicate an infection that way and there is a risk that an allergy may develop to something in the cream.

The best treatment is the simplest. Just cover the boil with a dry dressing and leave it alone to come to a head and burst.

If you want to speed up the process and relieve the pain at the same time then a little gentle heat will do as much good as anything. If the boil is in an accessible place put a well wrapped hot water bottle on top of the dressing. If the boil is in an inaccessible place (such as on an eyelid) wrap a piece of clean lint or cotton around a spoon, dip the material into a bowl of hot water and then hold it a few inches away from the site of the boil.

Once a boil has burst it is vital to remember that the stuff that comes out is extremely infectious. It is a mixture of live and dead cells and bacteria. If you are not careful the bacteria will infect more sweat glands, hair follicles and sebaceous glands and you will soon be dealing with a crop of boils.

To make sure that no extra boils develop you must clean around the area very carefully with soap and water or with a liquid antiseptic. There is still no need to use antiseptic creams or ointments. Change the dressing on the boil every few hours while it is discharging and be careful to burn the old dressings as soon as you can. Don't just dump them into the waste bin.

If, despite all your precautions, additional boils develop you should seek medical advice. If you have cleaned the skin round the original boil then the most likely explanation is that someone in the family has a store of bacteria on deposit somewhere. To find that store your doctor will have to take some swabs and send them to the laboratory. The organisms responsible for boils often live in the nose (which is why your doctor will probably want to take nasal swabs from everyone in the family). Once the laboratory has identified the carrier then he or she can be treated—probably with an antibiotic.

The other reason for seeing the doctor if a crop of boils develop is that he will need to check the urine for sugar. Diabetes mellitus is a condition which tends to make the development of boils more likely and although the risk is fairly slight it is a disorder which must be excluded.

There are three specific conditions when you should seek medical advice where boils, carbuncles and styes are concerned.

1   If a boil or carbuncle becomes very large, very painful or doesn't look as though it is going to burst by itself your doctor may need to incise the boil with a clean scalpel blade and drain out the infected contents.

2   If a boil is in a difficult position or is dangerously close to some easily damaged organ (for example close to the eye or the ear or a joint) then you should get your doctor to look at it.

3   A doctor's advice should be sought if red lines appear on the skin around a boil. These red lines suggest that an infection isn't being contained within the boil but is spreading through the surrounding skin. When this happens an antibiotic may be needed to prevent the infection causing additional problems.

BREASTS

Facts about breast lumps and advice on how you can examine your own breasts

Up to the age of 20 breast cancer is virtually unheard of. Between 20 and 30 more than 99% of breast lumps are harmless. But between the ages of 30 and 60 one in twenty women will develop breast cancer. Breast cancer is one of the commonest causes of death among women—particularly those between the ages of 35 and 54.

The main symptom is usually a lump—most commonly in

the upper, outer quarter of the breast. The lump, usually pain-less, is invariably easier to feel than to see. Other symptoms include changes in the nipple.

It is now known that:

● Breast cancer tends to run in families.

● Women who have never had children are most at risk of developing breast cancer.

● A high protein, high fat diet increases the risk of breast cancer.

● Women who are overweight are more at risk.

● A high fibre diet reduces the risk of breast cancer.

A few years ago the standard treatment for breast cancer was complete removal of the breast. Today, however, most surgeons believe that removing just the tumour—rather than the whole breast—produces just as good a survival rate.

In those relatively rare cases where breast removal is consid-ered essential the missing breast can be reconstructed artificially—sometimes at the same time as the removal opera-tion is performed.

Here are two facts that should encourage any woman who finds a lump in a breast:

1   No less than 98% of breast lumps that measure less than half an inch across and which are discovered by women exam-ining themselves do *not* require any disfiguring surgery.

2   When a breast lump does turn out to be cancerous women who have found their own lump have a survival rate 50% higher than other women.

Every woman should examine her own breasts regularly—preferably once a week or once a month. Indeed, figures show that despite huge expenditure on screening equipment 90% of breast cancer is discovered by women themselves.

Women should:

● Check the shape and outline of their breasts for any obvious lumps

● Observe their nipples—looking for changes, bleeding, discharge or inversion

● Physically examine themselves once a month—preferably

just after a menstrual period when their breasts are usually at their softest.

Follow this set examination plan to reduce the risk of missing any area:

1   Undress to your waist and sit or stand in front of a mirror. Let your hands hang loosely by your sides. Look for any changes in the size or appearance of your breasts or nipples. Look for any puckering or dimpling of the skin and check your nipples for any bleeding or discharge.

2   Lie down. Remember that both breasts will have a soft, general lumpiness because of fat and milk producing glands. Both breasts should feel much the same.

3   Put your left hand under your head. Examine your left breast with your right hand. Use the flat of your fingers, not the tips. Begin by examining the inner half of your breast and gradually working your way towards the nipple.

4   Bring your left arm down to your side and examine the other, outer half of your breast in the same way. Feel in your armpit too, looking for any lumps there.

5   Examine your right breast in exactly the same way—but using your left hand.

6   If you find anything unusual or worrying make a mental note of where the lump or change is and make an appointment to see your doctor as soon as possible. In the meantime, try not to keep feeling the lump—its best to leave it alone. Remember that few breast lumps are cancerous and that those which are can be treated much more effectively if found early.

If you don't know how to examine your breasts see your own GP and ask him to tell you what to feel for—and how to do it.

BROKEN BONES

See Fractures

BURNS

7 tips for dealing with them

Cold water is the best treatment for a burn—it may hurt a little but it will prevent blistering and will minimise the amount of damage that is done. The burnt area should be kept under water for at least five minutes.

Here are some other tips for dealing with burns.

1   Always get medical advice for anything other than a very small, superficial burn.

2   If a burn involves a finger or hand remove all rings and bracelets if you can. The tissues may swell making later removal difficult.

3   *Don't* put any cream, grease or oil onto a burn. It is a myth that you should smear butter onto a burn. Don't put anything other that a clean, dry dressing onto a burn.

4   *Don't* try picking off bits of burnt clothing—leave that for the experts to do later.

5   *Don't* touch the burnt area more than you have to.

6   *Don't* burst any blisters.

CANCER

10 ways to help fight cancer and win

Cancer is, without doubt, the most feared word in the language.

Most people don't even like to say or read the word and as a result there are dozens of myths and misconceptions about it.

The commonest and most destructive myth is that cancer always kills. It doesn't. Between a third and a half of all those who get cancer recover—usually living long, perfectly healthy, perfectly normal lives.

The second major myth is that cancer is one disease. It isn't. Cancer is a disease created by deformed or damaged cells. There are scores of different types of cell in your body and so there are scores of different types of cancer. Over 200 in fact.

With so many different types of cancer there are, of course, many different types of treatment. But there are some things that *all* cancer patients can do to help themselves.

1   Make up your mind that you are going to fight. A study of women with breast cancer showed conclusively that women with a fierce will to live were twice as likely to survive as those who were pessimistic.

2   Spend as much time as you can with people you like and people who make you laugh. There is no doubt now that laughter can help defeat a whole range of serious disorders—including cancer.

3   Assert yourself. If you are in hospital and the doctors and nurses won't tell you what you want to know, make a fuss and make a nuisance of yourself until they answer your questions. People who stand up for themselves stand a much better chance of surviving.

4   Build up your self confidence. Learn to respect and value yourself. Think of all your good qualities and strengths. People who develop and die of cancer often have a low opinion of themselves.

5   Don't be afraid to show your emotions. If you feel angry let your anger out. If you want to cry, then cry. Share your emotions—the more you store them up the more damage you'll do.

6   Learn to relax.

7   Eat a good, healthy diet containing as much natural food as possible. Fresh fruit and vegetables are much better than pre–packaged foods.

8   Join up with other people suffering from the same condition. There are scores of self–help groups—your doctor should be able to put you in touch.

9   Use the power of your mind to combat your cancer. Think of your cancer cells as bad guys and your body's defence

cells as good guys. Imagine your body's defences fighting and destroying frightened cancer cells. This sort if imagery really does work!

10 Learn as much as you can about your disease. Ignorance breeds fear and anxiety.

CATARRH

A quick but effective remedy

A menthol inhalation is the best way to clear the sinuses and relieve the stuffiness and headaches associated with catarrh. Put one small menthol crystal (you can buy a bottle full from the chemist quite cheaply) into a bowl of hot water and then breathe in the rising vapour. Do this a couple of times a day and you should find that you get relief from your symptoms quite quickly. Incidentally, you will also find that you'll benefit if you keep out of smoke filled rooms. Cigarette smoke makes catarrh much worse.

CHEST PAIN

Most people associate chest pain with heart disease but there are very many other causes of pain in the chest—most of which are commoner than heart pain. The majority of incidents of chest pain are relatively harmless—though all cases of chest pain should be investigated by a doctor.

Common causes of pains in the chest include indigestion and chest infection.

Stress and anxiety is probably one of the commonest causes of chest pain.

Other possible causes include: broken ribs (due to a fall), strained muscles (following exercise or a sudden movement), and nerve irritation (caused by osteoarthritis or a disorder of the vertebrae).

The treatment will, of course, depend upon the underlying cause of the pain.

CHICKENPOX

To begin with the spots caused by the chickenpox virus look like small pimples. Within a day or so they gradually grow into blisters which obviously contain fluid. The spots can start just about anywhere on the body but they usually begin on the head. They can occur inside the mouth where they are particularly painful. The chest and abdomen tend to be more severely affected than the arms and legs.

Chickenpox spots continue to arrive for three or four days and this means that at any one time there will be spots present in several stages of development. It is rarely possible to make a diagnosis before the spots become clearly visible although just before the characteristic rash appears the sufferer will usually complain of a headache and may have a fever and an indistinct blotchy rash.

Chickenpox is very infectious. It is spread by touch or breath. After contact with an infected individual it may be two or three weeks before symptoms develop. A patient with chickenpox will be infectious from twenty-four hours before the spots appear until the spots have all turned into dried scabs. The scabs themselves are not infectious.

There is no cure for chickenpox. The commonest symptom associated with the disease is itching and this can often be best dealt with by an application of calamine lotion. If the patient scratches too much permanent scars can develop, so it is important to alleviate itching as much as possible. The damage done by night time scratching can be minimised by wearing gloves or mittens.

If the itching is very bad there is a risk that the spots will become infected. So, if calamine doesn't help ask your doctor for assistance. He may, for example, prescribe an antihistamine to help dampen down the need to scratch.

A patient with chickenpox should be quite well apart from the itchy rash. If there are other symptoms it is important to get in touch with the doctor quickly since there can be complications. Vomiting, headaches and sleeplessness are three of the most important symptoms to watch out for.

CHILDREN AND TV

Does your child watch too much TV?

The average child watches at least four hours of television a day. But there is a growing amount of evidence to show that watching too much TV could ruin his health.

Here are some of the ways in which your child's health can be damaged by television.

1   Everybody needs exercise. You don't get any exercise watching television. It is fair enough to let children spend the day in front of the television set if it is raining. But if it is dry encourage them to play outside more often.

2   Many children slump in front of the television set in a position that is terrible for their spines. Back pain and muscle aches are the long term consequence of this. If your child seems stiff or uncomfortable after watching TV then he needs a firmer chair. Or persuade him to use cushions or, even, a special back support.

3   Sitting too close to the television can produce eyestrain and headaches. Don't let children crouch on the floor right in front of the television set. They should be sitting at least six feet from the set—and preferably further away.

4   Don't have the volume turned up too high. Exposure to too much noise can cause deafness.

5   Eating while watching television is a common cause of indigestion and other stomach upsets. Try to fix television viewing so that your child isn't going to eat and watch TV at the same time. Use the video recorder if possible.

6   Watching horror movies can produce nightmares and sleep disturbances in children. Don't let children watch late night films unless you have vetted the films first.

7   People who watch TV indiscriminately often spend far too little time talking to one another. The result can be depression, loneliness and relationships that break down. When a group of 4 to 6 year olds were asked which they preferred—

daddy or television—around half said they preferred television.

8 Too much television destroys a child's imagination—and can damage creative skills.

9 Watching endless advertisements on television can make viewers feel frustrated and dissatisfied with their lives. Children who have hobbies and who play active sports are less likely to be adversely affected by what they see on television.

10 Don't let children watch news programmes alone. Television often frightens and worries sensitive viewers. A child who is upset by what he has seen on the screen may need comfort and reassurance—and explanations.

Do your children watch too much TV?

Answer these questions as honestly as you can:

1 Is the TV always on whenever your children are in the house?

2 Do your children make straight for the TV when they enter the house?

3 After sitting down to watch TV do your children watch straight through until it is time to go to bed or time to go out—or until you stop them?

4 Do your children frequently watch programmes which you would describe as rubbish?

5 Do your children have TV sets in their bedrooms?

6 Do your children usually work or eat while watching TV?

7 Would your children be terribly upset if the TV broke down and couldn't be mended for 48 hours?

8 Do your children watch more than 20 hours of TV a week?

9 If you are booking a holiday do your children ask about the availability of a TV?

10 Do your children every say 'Ssshhh!' if you speak while they are watching a TV programme?

11 Do your children read less than you would like them to?

12 Do your children talk about TV characters as though they were real?

If you have answered YES to any of these questions then your children are probably TV addicts. This may sound like a joke. It isn't. If your children are TV addicts you should try to cut down their viewing. You may need to do it slowly. It will probably be as painful as controlling any addiction. Encourage your children to take up hobbies and sports, to start playing games and reading books. Play with them to encourage them!

☞ *See also* Electricity.

CHILDREN STARTING SCHOOL

How to make it easy for your child

Your child's first day at school is an important day in his life— as well as yours. But if you know what to expect then you can ensure that it is an exciting, happy day rather than a traumatic, tearful day. You can ensure that it is a day to look back on with happiness rather than a day that creates numerous problems for the future.

First, and most important of all, do remember that your child's attitude towards starting school will be coloured by your attitudes.

If you spend a lot of time telling your child 'not to worry' and assuring them that 'everything will be fine' then they will be bound to worry. That is just simple human nature.

Take your child to the school gates and stand there with tears in your eyes and your child will enter the classroom with tears in his eyes too.

If, however, you are positive and enthusiastic then your child will be positive and enthusiastic. Tell him that you are looking forward to the *big day* and that it is going to be very exciting and he will look forward to it too.

I have known children get as excited and enthusiastic about starting school as they have been about going to a party or to the seaside.

When children start school in a flood of tears it is usually because of an attitude they have acquired from their parents. Tell your child that you want to know what happens and you want to be told all about it. Tell them that it is going to be an adventure—and your child will start school with enthusiasm.

Attitude is the most important factor in ensuring that your child's introduction to school life is joyful rather than painful, happy rather than miserable.

But there are many other things that you can do.

You should try to arrange for your child to look inside the school before he starts attending in earnest. After all it is the strangeness of the place that is part of the day. Let your child get used to the fact that the furniture is different, the decorations are different and the plumbing is different and you will have got rid of several possible sources of anxiety.

Given a chance to study these surroundings with their parents most children find the specially built chairs and tables and the low slung washbasins tremendous fun.

Let your child take a little piece of home to school with him. Homesickness is one of the major problems for youngsters starting school for the first time, so let your child take a small and favourite toy—something that he can put into his pocket or satchel; something that he can take out and hold whenever he feels particularly lonely and vulnerable.

Next, try to make sure that nothing changes at home during those first days at school.

If one parent is going to start work when he or she has been at home then, if possible, delay it for a week or two after the child has started school. Children starting school need security, comfort and continuity at home. They need to feel that every-thing at home is stable and unchanging.

If you are normally out at work, make one small change: try to arrange to get time off work so you can meet your child when school finishes. Someone will have to meet him, of course, but it is best if it is someone really close to him: someone he knows and loves. He will also want to be able to tell you about all the exciting things that have happened to him.

You can also help by asking around your neighbours to find out whether there are any other local children starting at the same school on the same day. If there are then arrange a meeting so that the children can all make friends. It is a lot easier to go into a new building if you recognise a few familiar faces.

Make sure that you find out in advance about what your child is expected to wear at school. If all the other children will be wearing some easily identifiable item of clothing then try to make sure that your child fits in. Nothing worries children more than standing out and looking different. (This may change when the child is older. But at school starting age it is fairly universal).

If children are allowed to wear whatever they like then make sure that your child starts school in something comfortable. Don't send him out in his best clothes with strict instructions not to get messy or dirty. If you do, that will be just another stress to be added to the pile.

Finally, do be prepared for the fact that your child's behaviour may be a little unusual when he comes home from school after that first day. He may be exceptionally noisy, he may feel tired and sleep, he may cry a little, he may want lots of love and cuddles, he may behave in a very babyish manner. All these are normal reactions to a very exceptional day.

CHOKING

Life saving techniques

There can be few things worse than watching someone choke to death because you don't know what to do.

This technique is suitable for adults and older children:

1   Get the person who is choking to stand. Get friends to help you drag him into an upright position.

2   Stand behind him with your arms round his waist.

3   Make a fist with your right hand and put your fist right in the middle of his tummy—between the bottom of his ribs and the top of his trousers.

4   Take hold of your fist with your other hand.

5   Press very firmly into his tummy. Pull inwards and upwards and really pull hard. You need a lot of pressure quite quickly.

By putting pressure on his abdomen you put pressure on his diaphragm. That, in turn, means that the pressure inside his chest will rise. And the increased pressure inside the chest will mean that any food obstructing the windpipe will be forced out quite rapidly. The obstruction will shoot out from the victim's throat like a bullet from a rifle.

If the technique doesn't work, do it again.

You can't use this life saving technique on small children, but for them there is an alternative.

Simply hold the child upside down (hanging on to both his legs) and get someone else to smack him quite hard on the back.

That will usually dislodge the obstruction.

This life saving technique is easy to learn and easy to do.

If someone really is choking to death there isn't any point in waiting for the doctor to come. By the time he arrives it will be too late.

CHOLESTEROL

Cholesterol, which is present in all animal tissues, has some similar properties to fat but is recognised as being potentially dangerous because if the level of cholesterol in your blood reaches too high a concentration, it can increase your chances of having a heart attack.

Cholesterol is present in many ordinary foods (cheese, chocolate, cream, eggs, heart, kidneys, liver, crab, lobster, brains, caviar) but most of the cholesterol in our bodies comes not from foods that contain cholesterol itself but from other fatty foods.

Our bodies can make their own cholesterol from saturated fats so if your diet contains a high quantity of saturated fat then your body will make more cholesterol and your blood cholesterol level will probably rise.

COLDS AND FLU

7 tips to help you stay healthy & 5 tips to help you fight colds and flu

Pop into your local pharmacy and you will see a huge range of expensive products designed to help you and your family stay cold and flu free during the winter. But I doubt if any of those products are worth buying. Despite all the claims there just are not any magic remedies that you can buy to keep cold or flu bugs at bay. The claims for products such as vitamin C have, I fear, been wildly exaggerated—unless you are actually deficient.

But here are seven tips that will help you and your family stay healthy—and five tips to help you deal with the symptoms of a cold (or flu) if the worst comes to the worst!

To PREVENT COLDS AND FLU

1   Don't turn your heating up too much. The bigger the difference between the temperature inside your house and the temperature outside the greater the shock to your system when you go out.

2   Make sure that everyone wears warm clothes when they go outside. Coats are essential, of course, but hats. scarves and gloves are also very important. And make sure that your family take their outdoor clothes off whenever they go indoors.

3   Don't let the air in your home get too dry. Catarrh and sinus problems commonly occur when there isn't enough moisture in the air. It may help to put bowls of water near to fires or radiators.

4   Make sure that everyone eats a good healthy diet. And a good breakfast is essential. Food provides the fuel that you need to keep your body's central heating system working.

5   Try to persuade everyone in your family *not* to touch their eyes. Researchers have shown that cold germs are usually transmitted by touch and often get into the body through the eyes. Hands will inevitably get infected but keep them

away from the eyes and you'll reduce the risk of infection.

6   Keep a little salt in the bathroom and at the first sign of a sore throat have a salt water gargle. It will do you just as much good as any of the more expensive gargles and mouthwashes.

7   Try to make sure that you know how to relax. Scientists have shown that people who worry a lot get more colds and flu than other people.

To treat colds and flu

1   The stuffed up feeling that often accompanies a cold can be best relieved with a good, old fashioned inhalation. Just pour some hot (not boiling) water into a bowl, add a menthol crystal (bought from your local pharmacy) and let the patient breathe in the medicated steam as it rises. Put a towel over his head if you like to help keep the vapour in the right place. Younger children who can't be helped in this way will feel better if you simply boil the kettle and let the vapour fill the air. You can help relieve the stuffed up feeling that keeps children awake by putting a small dab of a mentholated balm on the child's chest.

2   Also try a hot lemon drink. Slice five lemons into two pints of cold water and add two tablespoonfuls of sugar or honey. Bring the mixture to the boil and simmer, reducing the liquid slightly. Then allow it all to cool. Afterwards add hot water to the concentrate as and when you need it. If you serve it in a large glass and persuade the patient to sniff the rising vapour before drinking, the lemon drink can be used as an inhalant and a soothing remedy for an irritated throat.

3   The best remedy for the aches and pains of flu is soluble aspirin (though aspirin is not suitable for children, of course) or paracetamol.

4   If you get a cold at a difficult time you can keep the symptoms at bay for a while by telling yourself that you are going to stay well. Your body will fight off the cold and give you a few days before the symptoms get really bad.

5   If any symptoms worry you or persist for five days or more then see your doctor. But don't be upset if he doesn't prescribe an antibiotic. Drugs like penicillin aren't any good for colds or flu.

COLD SORES

Cold sores are small blisters around the mouth caused by the herpes simplex virus. Most people are infected by the HSV 1 virus which causes cold sores. Usually the virus lies dormant in nerve cells but it is occasionally reactivated—causing cold sores. Exposure to cold winds or sunshine may trigger an attack of cold sores—as may an infection or tiredness. Cold sores are itchy and they irritate. They usually disappear within a week or so. If developing cold sores are seen early enough a doctor can prescribe an anti viral drug.

COLIC

The word colic simply means a cramp–like abdominal pain that comes and goes. Colic commonly affects babies between 2 weeks and 3 months of age. It often goes on for several months and then disappears as mysteriously as it came. Many babies suffer badly from it; it usually starts in the early evening and often lasts for hours. The baby who has colic will cry, clench his fists, pull his legs up, scream occasionally and go quite red.

There are lots of possible explanations. Colic may be caused by wind. Some doctors claim it can be caused by something in cow's milk. And a few doctors claim that babies get colic when their mothers are under stress.

If your baby develops colic you should call your doctor for advice. If he says there isn't anything he can do, try to stay as relaxed as possible. If you are giving your baby cow's milk, it might be worth trying to wean him off it. In my view, gripe waters and special colic remedies are a waste of money.

The main consolation I can offer is that most babies grow out of the colic by the time they reach 6 months of age.

CONJUNCTIVITIS

The conjunctiva is the thin membrane that covers the surface of the eye. If this becomes irritated the condition is known as conjunctivitis. The usual cause is an infection although foreign bodies can also produce irritation which can lead to inflammation. Allergic reactions can also produce conjunctivitis.

It is important to be aware of the various possible causes of conjunctivitis so that you can deal effectively with the source of the problem (though remember that conjunctivitis should always be seen by a doctor as soon as possible—as should all eye problems).

When conjunctivitis is due to an allergy reaction, the symptoms will usually be itching, watering, redness and swelling around the eye.

When the conjunctivitis is due to an infection, the eye will often be sticky and 'gritty'. This feeling is often worse in the morning. There may also be a yellow discharge of pus that can result in the eyelids being stuck together in the morning. If this happens they should be bathed and gently prised apart.

This type of infective conjunctivitis is itself very infectious and care should be taken not to spread the infection around. The sufferer should use disposable towels and avoid rubbing the eyes.

Conjunctivitis produced by causes other than infection is not contagious.

Preventing non–infectious conjunctivitis is fairly easy—you have to locate the allergy and eliminate or reduce its contact with the eye.

If you feel that conjunctivitis is caused by an infection then you should see your doctor who can prescribe antibiotic drops or ointment. There can often be a sensitivity to light associated with conjunctivitis so wearing dark glasses may help.

Always seek medical advice immediately if you notice any loss of vision or if you feel any pain in or around the eye. You should also see your doctor straight away if you suspect that a foreign body may be causing the conjunctivitis.

CONSTIPATION
Ways to deal with it

Many people feel that if their bowels are not opened and emptied as regularly as post boxes then there is something wrong. The bowels of thousands of individuals (including babies and children) are regularly attacked with powerful laxatives when there is, in truth, nothing wrong with them.

For most children the frequency with which the bowels are opened is of no significance. Just because nothing is passed for a day or two doesn't mean that the child is constipated. Much more important is the nature and consistency of the stool that is passed. Small, hard stools that can only be passed with difficulty, discomfort and great effort are good evidence that your child is suffering from constipation.

The single most important cause of constipation involves the diet. With bowels you can only get out what you put in. The relationship to diet is particularly important with babies who are much more likely to suffer from constipation if they are bottle fed than if they are breast fed. Constipation is, indeed, extremely rare among breast fed babies. Breast milk is the perfect formula for most babies and there is very little waste in it. A breast fed baby can go for a week without a bowel movement and still be perfectly healthy.

Among bottle fed babies constipation is slightly more common and when it does occur it is usually the result of the diet. Using too much milk powder is a common cause. Adding more water (or perhaps even including a feed of dilute fruit juice) will usually clear up the problem. If it does not do the job then the constipation may have simply have been produced by the fact that the baby is being underfed.

When these simple remedies don't work or if the constipation is accompanied by pain or any other worrying symptom then it is obviously important to seek medical advice straight away. By itself constipation is not a health hazard but it can, quite rarely, be a sign of an underlying disorder which requires professional treatment. It is very uncommon for a baby's constipation to be caused by anything more than a dietary imbalance. However, the straining that may accompany severe constipation can produce a split or fissure around the anus and the pain from that can itself cause an unwillingness to open the bowels.

When constipation occurs among slightly older children it may be a result of shyness or embarrassment. Children often get constipated because they find school lavatories cold, dirty, smelly or lacking in essential privacy. The same reasons often explain why children get constipated on holiday (particularly if they are camping). It is also worth remembering that toddlers who are under pressure from their parents to 'perform' may sometimes rebel and deliberately refuse to cooperate. When that happens the best remedy is to take the pressure off and leave things alone for a while.

I don't think laxatives should ever be given to children without a doctor's authority. Constipation in a child is usually the result of a dietary problem, a psychological problem or some underlying physical abnormality. There is no place for laxatives. Indeed, laxatives can make constipation worse—and into a long term problem.

To deal with constipation in a toddler, child or adult I would recommend plenty of fluids, lots of fruit, a good supply of fresh fruit juice, wholemeal bread, wholemeal cereal and green vegetables. Milk, biscuits, sweets and cake are all likely to make things worse. As with most problems which are related to diet a well balanced diet is the long term solution.

CONVULSIONS AND FITS IN CHILDREN
10 practical tips

The natural fear and anxiety a parent feels when he or she sees his or her child having a fit is often made worse because they don't know what is happening, what they can do about it and what the likely consequences might be.

Convulsions are an involuntary spasm or contraction of the

muscles. There may be a single spasm or a series of spasms. A fit is the same thing as a convulsion and the words are interchangeable.

The human brain is filled with millions of electrical connections and with the aid of electrical impulses messages travel to and fro. Those electrical impulses carry information in from sensory organs such as the eyes and ears and send messages out to the organs and muscles around the body. If you see a car coming towards you, your eyes pass the information on to your brain by means of electrical impulses and your brain then uses more electricity to contract the muscles needed to help you jump out of the way.

If for any reason there is a sudden, abnormal burst of electrical activity within the brain all the pathways which were up until that moment filled with normal impulses carrying messages to and fro will be overwhelmed. The result will be that muscles all over the body will be stimulated to act in no particular order and in no logical sequence. The muscles of the legs can twitch, eyelid muscles can flutter and the arms may fly all over the place. The muscles which control the function of the bladder and bowel may be affected. Breathing may stop temporarily as the chest muscles are affected and your child may go unconscious. That is a convulsion and the unusual muscle activity is simply a sign that there has been some sort of electrical storm inside the brain.

There is no pain accompanying this mixture of symptoms and your child will not be aware of what is happening. Afterwards he won't remember anything about it. Once a convulsion has finished your child will probably fall asleep and rest calmly and peacefully. Convulsions tend to affect parents more than they affect children.

So, what causes this electrical storm?

No one really knows exactly what goes on inside the human brain.

What we do know, however, is that all sorts of different things can trigger a fit and children and babies seem to be particularly susceptible. The electrical bursts which cause the fits can be produced in many ways. A low blood sugar can produce a fit and a frustrated or thwarted child who is having a breath holding attack can have a convulsion but the commonest cause is a high temperature (known as febrile convulsions in young children).

It is pretty safe to say that if you have a child aged between six months and five years of age and he has a high temperature and a convulsion then the two are probably linked.

One in 25 children aged between 6 months and 5 years old will have a convulsion or fit because of a fever.

In the development of a febrile convulsion it is the speed with which the temperature rises that is more important than the temperature itself. A sudden rise of a few degrees is more likely to produce a convulsion than a slow steady rise to a higher temperature. So, to prevent a febrile convulsion keep an eye on your child's temperature. If it seems to be rising fast take off some of his clothes, open the window and turn off the heating. Call the doctor straight away. Tepid sponging helps a lot. Just dip a sponge or cloth in a bowl of lukewarm water and wipe gently over his skin. Give lots of fluids but don't give other medicines unless they have been specifically prescribed for your child.

Children who have one febrile convulsion are more likely to have a second but the likelihood of a child having a second convulsion falls as he gets older. If there is a family history of febrile convulsions there does seem to be a greater chance of a child having a convulsion.

There is a lot of confusion about the difference between a convulsion and an epileptic fit. The confusion is made worse by the fact that epilepsy isn't a single disease at all but is the rather woolly name given to all disorders which produce convulsions and a loss of consciousness. In practice most people use the word epilepsy to refer to fits which recur, usually without there being any obvious explanation. If I had my way the word epilepsy would be hidden away in the medical dictionary where no one could find it. Fits are either isolated or recurrent. Most children who have convulsions have one and no more.

You may suspect epilepsy but you should not try to make a diagnosis yourself—see your doctor.

In the meantime, if anyone in your presence has a fit here is what you should do.

1   Try not to panic. Most convulsions will do no lasting harm. I know that advice may sound trite but there is a lot you can do and so you should stay calm.

2   Lie your child on the floor on his right side. Turn his face towards the floor so that if he vomits he won't choke or inhale any vomit. Your child will be safest on the floor because he won't have anywhere to fall.

3   Loosen any tight clothing. Do not put a spoon or any other object in his mouth. People do this so that the person having the fit doesn't bite his tongue. However, a spoon tends to be rather hard and the result is often that instead of ending up with a bitten tongue (which will heal) the patient ends up with broken teeth (which won't).

4   Move furniture and other hard objects out of the way so that he won't hurt himself by banging into things.

5   If he has a high temperature try to cool him. Remove any clothing that you can undo easily. Open a window or turn on a fan. Use a sponge or cloth soaked in tepid water to wipe him down. Don't use a cold sponge because that will make things worse by closing down some of the body's temperature control mechanisms.

6   Make sure that he doesn't swallow his tongue. If necessary pull the tongue forward.

7   Telephone the doctor to let him know what is happening and ask his advice. Most convulsions last less than five minutes so he is unlikely to get to you before it is all over.

8   Don't give anything to eat or drink during or immediately after a fit. And don't try giving any medicines unless he has had previous convulsions and your doctor has given you specific drugs with specific instructions. If the fit lasts for more than 5 or 10 minutes and the doctor is not on the way then you should take the patient to the nearest casualty

department. He will probably stop fitting before you get there but he might just need an injection to help control the convulsion. Talk to your doctor about the fit afterwards and ask him to make a diagnosis about the cause of the convulsion. If your doctor is uncertain about what caused the fit he may arrange for hospital tests. If he thinks that your child has an infection he may prescribe an antibiotic.

9 Hold the victim if you like but do not restrain him and never try physically to prevent a fit or convulsion.

10 Ignore anyone who suggests putting your child into a bath of cold water or who advocates artificial respiration. Children are more likely to be harmed by the inappropriate treatment than by convulsions.

Convulsions may be frightening for the onlooker but they are usually harmless. A study of over 1,700 children who had convulsions showed no lasting damage as a result of the fits. There is no link between an isolated convulsion and brain damageand it is not true that a child who has had an isolated convulsion is likely to develop recurrent fits in later life.

☞ *See also* Epilepsy.

COT DEATH

6 tips to keep your baby safe

Cot Death Syndrome—officially and more accurately known as Sudden Infant Death Syndrome (SIDS) since not all such deaths occur in the baby's cot—is, in many countries, now the commonest cause of death among children aged between one week and two years.

Every year thousands of sets of parents will lose an apparently healthy baby to this mysterious and much feared killer disease. The term 'cot death' was coined in 1954 to describe unexpected deaths for which no adequate explanation could be found. Since 1971, when SIDS was first recognised as an 'official' cause of death, the number of babies succumbing to this mystery disease has increased steadily.

During the last decade and a half, dozens of eminent researchers have struggled—but failed—to find a completely satisfactory explanation. The confusion and the lack of knowledge means that parents often blame themselves.

Typically, a baby is put into its cot at night to sleep and found dead when the parents wake in the morning. Often parents feel that the finger of suspicion is pointing at them. They wonder if friends or relatives are blaming them for their baby's death.

So what does cause SIDS?

If there is a single cause then it's something—a strange virus perhaps—that medical scientists still haven't managed to identify.

My view is that it is more likely that SIDS are caused by a number of different disorders.

Here are some of the possible explanations that have been put forward:

1   Infection.

Babies are as vulnerable to infection as you'd expect them to be. We are more vulnerable to infection than our ancestors. Inevitably babies suffer more than anyone.

2   Cow's milk.

Babies fed on cow's milk may die because of an allergy.

3   Whooping cough vaccine.

Many deaths occur shortly after a baby has been vaccinated against whooping cough. Coincidence? Maybe not.

4   Overheating.

Babies are vulnerable to heat as well as to cold. Sometimes parents pile too many bedclothes onto their baby to protect him against the cold—the result can then be that the baby's body overheats.

5   Tranquillisers.

It is known that SIDS are more common when mothers have taken addictive drugs during pregnancy. Tranquillisers are the commonest drugs used by pregnant women. Could the use of these drugs be killing babies?

Here are some facts that will help you find out whether—and when—your baby could be at risk.

1   SIDS is slightly commoner among boys than girls.

2   Many more babies die of this disease in winter than in summer. The peak months seem to be December and January.

3   Babies usually die of SIDS between 2 and 4 months of age, and nearly always before six months of age.

4   Breast fed babies are less at risk than bottle fed babies.

5   Having your baby in bed with you could be dangerous—babies are so small and delicate that they may be suffocated by tight bedclothes. But sleeping near to your baby—with your baby in the same room—may be helpful.

6   A mother who has lost one baby runs a higher risk of losing another—one woman lost 4 babies this way.

7   Very small babies are more at risk.

8   Twins are more at risk.

Here are some tips to help you keep your baby as safe as possible.

1   Try to keep the baby's room at a steady temperature of around 65 degrees Fahrenheit. A room that is too hot or too cold is dangerous. And don't use too many bedclothes.

2   Make sure that your baby's cot has a firm mattress. Don't give a baby a pillow.

3   Breastfeed if you can for the first few months of life. Breastfeeding helps protect your baby against infection. If you have to bottle feed follow the instructions carefully. Adding extra powder is dangerous.

4   Don't let anyone smoke in the same room as your baby. Smoking can increase the chances of chest infection developing.

5   If you think that your baby is especially at risk then talk to your doctor about obtaining a special breathing alarm—designed to alert you if your baby stops breathing.

6   Put your baby to sleep on his back or side—not on his stomach (unless your doctor has advised otherwise—there are *some* babies who should sleep on their stomachs).

COUGHING

The human body contains a large number of marvellous automatic defence mechanisms designed to protect its internal workings. One of these defence mechanisms is the cough reflex. If anything threatens to block the tubes leading down into the lungs a series of automatic responses are brought into action to deal with the threatened blockage.

In some circumstances the cough reflex can prove life saving. For example, the child who has a badly infected chest will be able to cough up material which might otherwise lie around in his lungs and make things worse. One of the problems doctors have to deal with when they are looking after patients who are deeply unconscious is that the cough reflex is absent. Without that vital reflex phlegm and mucus can collect in the lungs and infections such as pneumonia can develop.

The most dramatic type of cough is the one that is produced when some foreign object gets into the tubes leading down into the lungs. If a child who is otherwise well suddenly develops a cough, he may have inhaled a small object which is threatening to block part of a lung. This can happen when a child is playing with small objects and it is particularly likely to occur when children throw small sweets or peanuts up into the air and play at catching them in their mouths.

When this happens and the coughing produces the foreign body there isn't much need to do anything else. If however the coughing persists then urgent medical attention is needed.

The cough that frightens mothers most is probably the characteristic 'whoop' that gives whooping cough its name. This infection usually starts with the symptoms of an ordinary cold. Then the child starts coughing and breathing in air through a partially closed trachea. It is the air going through this closed windpipe that produces the 'whoop'. Vomiting is very common with whooping cough since small children are often unable to spit out phlegm. They bring it up just far enough to swallow and the accumulation of phlegm in the stomach then makes them vomit.

If you think that your child has whooping cough, you should get in touch with your doctor straight away.

Coughing can be and often is an entirely unnecessary and quite exhausting phenomenon. Coughs are common at night when mucus trickles down the back of the throat. This is common when someone has a cold or is suffering from catarrh. You may be able to deal with this either by sleeping on an extra pillow or by trying to sleep in a different position.

Night time coughs can also be caused by the fact that the temperature in the bedroom may be different from the temperature in the rest of the house. If you think this may be the case then it may help to put a heater on in the bedroom for an hour or so before bedtime. Just taking the chill out of the air is often all that is needed. If the room gets too hot and stuffy, on the other hand, that can also cause a night time cough.

The other very common cause of a ticklish, unproductive cough is cigarette smoke. A child who is breathing air which is thick with cigarette smoke is likely to acquire a permanent cough.

All these irritating coughs can be alleviated with the aid of a hot lemon drink that you can make yourself. Simply slice lemons into water, add honey and boil. When you serve the mixture just add water to taste. This will do as much good as any branded cough medicine or cough sweet that you can buy.

Finally, some people do acquire a coughing habit. Often a leftover from a cold or a chest infection, the cough becomes something of a nervous tic and can be most aggravating for everyone. As long as your doctor has confirmed that there is nothing to worry about just try to ignore it. If you make a fuss the cough is likely to last for longer.

☞ *See also* Whooping cough.

CRAMP

A simple remedy that works

People often wake up at night with cramp in their lower legs. The pains are usually thought to be caused by the collection of waste products in the muscles which have collected there because of poor circulation.

To avoid cramp make sure that your bedclothes are not too tight around your feet—and avoid wearing tight stockings, socks or garters.

And try this exercise:

● stand barefoot one yard away from a wall

● lean forwards until your hands touch the wall but keep your heels on the floor

● maintain this position for ten seconds and repeat it once

Do this exercise three times a day for a week and then nightly before going to bed.

CRYING IN BABIES

9 causes

There are hundreds of reasons why a baby or small child may start crying. Here are some of the commonest:

1 Hunger

As soon as children can talk they will tell you when they are hungry. Small babies can't tell you anything—so they cry. A baby who hasn't had enough milk at one feed will often wake and start crying an hour or so later.

2 Pain

A child in pain will often cry much louder than at any other time. Mothers (and fathers) can often tell when crying is caused by genuine physical pain.

3 Teething

Babies are sometimes irritable—and likely to cry—when they are teething

4   Loneliness

Babies who are bored or feel that they have been ignored for too long will often start crying. Babies need all the love and comfort they can get—crying is sometimes just a way of reminding you that they are there!

5   Colic

Some experts believe that colic is caused by wind. Others argue that colicky pains develop when a baby is aware that his parents are under stress.

6   Discomfort

A baby who is cold, wet or in a draught will often cry to draw attention to his problem. Solve his problem and he'll stop crying.

7   Illness

Crying is often an early and very non specific symptom of illness. A child who cries may be sickening for something— or may already have something.

8   Sadness

Babies and children can get depressed and miserable just as easily as adults.

9   Tiredness

A baby who is tired will often cry a lot.

Don't be shy about asking for your doctor's advice if your baby is crying. Crying—particularly if it is accompanied by other symptoms—may be an important sign of an underlying problem.

CYSTITIS

Including 7 tips to help you conquer cystitis

Cystitis—an inflammation of the bladder—is an extremely common problem for women. Eight out of ten suffer from it occasionally, repeatedly or even constantly. It is commoner among women than men because the female urethra (the tube that carries urine down from the bladder) is much shorter and more vulnerable to infection than the male urethra.

The two symptoms most commonly associated with cystitis are: pain on passing urine and having to pass small amounts of urine unusually frequently. Other symptoms include the passing of cloudy, discoloured or blood stained urine.

Cystitis after sex is sometimes called 'honeymoon' cystitis because brides are supposed to be exceptionally vulnerable to it. There are two reasons why a woman is likely to get cystitis after sex. First, her partner might give her an infection. Second, her urethra runs close to the vagina and is easily bruised.

Women can minimise the chances of picking up an infection by making sure both that they and their partner wash before sex and that they empty their bladder after sex. It is possible to minimise the chances of trauma to your urethra by experimenting with different positions. And a woman can also help herself by avoiding aggressive thrusting or deep penetration; by placing a pillow under her bottom if she makes love in the missionary position and by making sure that her vagina is well lubricated before sex.

Here's some general advice for cystitis sufferers:

1   Whenever you need to pass urine try and do so as soon as you can. If you delay too long then you may make your problem worse.

2   Cystitis can be caused or made worse by concentrated fruit juices, acid tasting fruits, sweet foods, spicy foods, tea, coffee and alcohol.

3   Drink huge amounts of plain water. Three or more pints a day are needed to help wash out the bladder and urethra. Cystitis sufferers who are already visiting the lavatory several times an hour may be reluctant to do this but it does help. You won't have to pass urine any more often but you will pass a greater quantity and that will help to wash out any bugs which are there.

4   The bugs that cause cystitis prefer acidic urine. In an emergency you can make your urine slightly alkaline by drinking

a solution of one teaspoonful of sodium bicarbonate (bicarbonate of soda) in water every three or four hours. Don't do this for more than one day. Talk to your pharmacist for advice about other ways to turn your urine alkaline.

5 When wiping yourself always wipe from front to back.

6 All you ever need when washing yourself around your vulva is warm water and a soft towel. Deodorants and antiseptics can cause more problems than they cure.

7 If the symptoms of cystitis persist for more than a day or two visit your doctor for a urine test. If any bugs can be identified a suitable antibiotic can be prescribed.

DERMATITIS

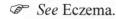 *See* Eczema.

DIABETES
10 practical tips

Under normal circumstances the pancreas gland produces a substance called insulin which is used in the body for the breakdown of sugar. When the production of insulin is impaired the body's ability to deal effectively with sugar is reduced. Diabetes mellitus or sugar diabetes is the name given to this disorder.

When diabetes develops in adults it is often fairly mild and the condition can be dealt with either by limiting the amount of sugar in the diet or by using drugs which stimulate the pancreas to produce more insulin.

When diabetes develops in children it tends to be more serious. It is usually necessary to reduce the amount of sugar in the diet and give insulin by injection. The amounts of sugar and insulin given need to be adjusted so that the two are balanced precisely.

Here are ten tips for diabetics:

1 Always seek medical advice if you are ill—even if it is just an

attack of the flu or a small wound. Illnesses can affect blood sugar levels and wounds can get infected easily in diabetics.

2   Include a healthy proportion of fibre in your diet. Your doctor should be able to arrange for you to talk to a dietician to plan a good, regular diet.

3   Look after your feet. Inspect them regularly and keep them clean and dry and warm. Make sure that your shoes and socks fit well.

4   Don't change your eating habits without discussing things with your doctor.

5   Take special care with alcohol and don't take over the counter medicines without checking first with your doctor.

6   Make sure you do not put on excess weight. Obesity can make diabetes more likely—or more difficult to control.

7   Learn as much as you can about your condition.

8   Regular exercise is essential—but check with your doctor before starting an exercise programme.

9   Take good care of your teeth and gums. Diabetics are more susceptible to gum disease.

10 Try to keep the stress in your life under control. Stress can result in changes in blood sugar levels.

DIARRHOEA

Food is probably the commonest cause of diarrhoea. Too much fat or too much carbohydrate in a baby's diet can produce soft, yellow stools. An excess of sugar is another possible cause of diarrhoea. In older children fruit is a common culprit. If, after a fruit picking expedition, your child suddenly develops diarrhoea then you can bet whatever you like that too much fruit never found its way into the basket.

Infections can also cause diarrhoea—and are the commonest cause of the problem in adults. If the diarrhoea is accompanied by vomiting, gastro–enteritis is possible.

Food poisoning is another cause of diarrhoea which usually

causes vomiting as well. Some types of food poisoning are extremely virulent and will spread around homes and schools very easily. Chest and throat infections can occasionally produce bouts of diarrhoea.

Antibiotics can produce the same symptoms by interfering with the normal bacterial inhabitants of the intestinal tract. A patient already being treated with antibiotics may well develop diarrhoea as a side effect.

A patient who has abdominal pain as well as diarrhoea may have appendicitis. Remember that individuals who are constipated may occasionally develop diarrhoea as the stools slowly seep around the blockage.

Finally, it is important to remember that people can easily develop diarrhoea when they are frightened, anxious or under too much pressure.

Diarrhoea tends to be more dangerous for young children than for adults. The main risk for a child with diarrhoea is that he will lose fluids so quickly that he becomes dehydrated. Obviously, the worse the diarrhoea the greater the risk and, if a child has been vomiting too, then the hazards are even greater – simply because fluid is being lost from both ends of the gastro intestinal tract.

The best way to diagnose dehydration is probably to look at your child's skin. In a normal child the skin will be extremely elastic. Pick up a pinch of skin and then let go and the skin will go back to its original position almost instantaneously. In a dehydrated child the skin will be far less elastic. Pick up a pinch of skin and then let go and the skin will remain in a slightly pinched position for a few seconds.

More serious signs of dehydration are sunken eyes, a dry mouth and rapid breathing. These signs indicate that a child needs urgent medical attention.

You should ask for medical advice if an adult:

1. Has diarrhoea for more than 48 hours.
2. Has diarrhoea and vomiting for more than 24 hours.
3. Shows any signs of dehydration.
4. Passes any blood.

5. Suffers from recurrent bouts of diarrhoea
6. Has a fever together with diarrhoea.
7. Complains of pain.
8. Looks ill or weak.
9. Worries you.

If, with a baby, the problem seems to have been caused by a feeding problem then the solution will usually be pretty obvious. A change in the type of formula or the constitution of the mix may be the answer for bottle fed babies. Make sure that you are not preparing the feed wrongly and don't allow yourself to add an extra spoonful of powder or sugar.

To help prevent dehydration it is vital to keep up the fluid intake when any child has diarrhoea. Breast fed babies should be given extra feeds on the breast and bottle fed babies should be given extra feeds of water. While the diarrhoea persists it is probably wise to reduce the strength of all milk feeds. Older children should be encouraged to drink large quantities of water or fairly weak fruit squash. Your pharmacist will have special mixtures you can buy to make sure that your child doesn't get low on salt and other essential nutrients.

When diarrhoea is accompanied by vomiting then avoid giving anything at all by mouth apart from water.

There are all sorts of anti diarrhoeal medicines available although I am not too enthusiastic about any of them. Kaolin is the commonest constituent of the mixtures—the theory behind its use is that when given by mouth it absorbs toxic substances from the intestinal tract, increases the bulk of the stools and helps the body get rid of irritant substances. I'm not entirely convinced that it does any of these things to any really useful extent but kaolin alone isn't likely to do much harm. You should not, of course, give any medicine for diarrhoea until you have sought medical advice.

The only other treatment that might be worth trying is yoghurt. If the diarrhoea was caused by an antibiotic then the yoghurt may be useful because it may help to restock the body with the sort of bacteria which normally live in the bowel and stop potentially damaging bacteria from moving in. Antibiotics kill off those bacteria and leave the area open to invasion. Yoghurt helps to restore the natural balance.

Finally, I must mention holiday diarrhoea. If you are away from home and you even suspect that the drinking water isn't pure then do make sure that you drink only bottled water. And do remember that ice cubes too are made from water. Don't buy ice creams that haven't been made and wrapped by a reputable manufacturer, avoid freshly washed salads and fruit that you cannot peel yourself, and make sure that you clean your teeth with bottled water too.

Don't forget that over eating is, like infection, a common cause of diarrhoea among holidaymakers.

DOCTORS

How to get the best out of your doctor

Every week thousands of men and women put off going for a medical examination because they're too anxious or shy. But putting off a visit to the doctor because you're suffering from 'pre-examination nerves' could be dangerous.

Here's my advice on how to get the best out of a visit to the doctor.

1 Don't delay. If you have a problem which is worrying you make an appointment now to see your doctor as soon as possible. The longer you wait the more you'll worry—and the worse things could get. If you think your problem is urgent, insist on having an appointment today or tomorrow. If the receptionist claims that the doctor can't fit you in, ask for a home visit—the chances are high that a surgery appointment will suddenly become available.

2 Be prepared for a physical examination. Would you be happy if a car mechanic tried to repair your car without lifting the bonnet? Dress in clothes you can get in and out of quickly. Stockings are easier than tights. Zips are quicker than buttons. Don't wear underwear that is going to embarrass you.

3 Don't worry about embarrassing or shocking your doctor. There is nothing you can tell your doctor that will shock him or her. Every week thousands of men and women who have 'trouble down below' walk in to the surgery, complain of a minor skin rash or a swollen vein and walk out without saying what is really on their minds!

4 Make up your mind beforehand what you want to tell your doctor. Write down a list of your important signs, symptoms, complaints and worries. Women of childbearing age should take along details of their last few periods. If you have to hunt through your diary, you'll get flustered and forget other important things.

5 Decide in advance what questions you want to ask—and what you want your doctor to do. And remember it is part of your family doctor's job to explain things to you. If you've seen a hospital doctor and haven't understood what he's said, ask your doctor to interpret the medical jargon for you.

6 Don't be startled or offended by questions your doctor asks.

7 Write down everything your doctor tells you to do. Your doctor will write down what you tell him. It makes sense for you to write down what he tells you.

8 If at the end of the consultation you aren't happy, ask for a second opinion. If your doctor refuses point blank to refer you, then I suggest that you change doctors.

Dry skin

5 tips for making it feel soft again

Normal skin feels soft and smooth and looks pink because it is well supplied with water. If the superficial skin cells don't contain enough water, the skin will feel rough and hard and will look cracked and uncomfortable.

If you've got dry, cracked skin the chances are either that you spend a lot of time in a centrally heated or air–conditioned atmosphere or that frequent washing has removed your skin's natural oils which help to keep it smooth and supple.

You can make your skin feel soft again by following these tips:

1   Use a moisturising cream regularly. Despite its name a moisturising cream doesn't add moisture to your skin but it does preserve the moisture that the skin contains. The oilier or creamier your moisturiser the more it will protect you. Keep a pot by every sink in the house and use it whenever you have had your hands in water.

2   You can give your skin extra protection by using a barrier cream—the extra oil will help protect your skin from irritating substances.

3   Wear rubber gloves whenever you have to put your hands in water. Detergents, bleaches and other chemicals can harm your skin. Gloves will protect you.

4   Remember that spending too long in the bath can dry your skin. Showers are better than baths. If you prefer a bath try not to soak for more than 15 minutes. And don't add bubbles—they tend to dry the skin even more. Bath oils will help protect you.

5   Air–conditioning and central heating are a common cause of dry skin—they dry the air so much that your body loses moisture. So make sure that you don't let your home or office get too dry. If you don't have any control over the radiators make sure that there are bowls of water sitting around.

DYSLEXIA

Dyslexia is much commoner than most people think. Some experts claim that one in 25 children may suffer from it—others that as many as 1 in 5 may be dyslexic. The basic problem dyslexic children face is that they find it difficult to understand and use letters and words. As a result they are invariably slow to learn to read, write and spell.

You should suspect that your child might be dyslexic if:

- she/he gets confused when learning particular letters—often writing them down upside down or back to front
- she/he is good at other subjects (maths, for example) but terrible at languages and spelling
- she/he is physically rather clumsy

It is *not* true that dyslexic children are in any way subnormal mentally. They are normally of average or higher than average intelligence.

Dyslexia is caused by a minor fault in the brain that may have been inherited or may be a result of an injury or an illness that occurred before, during or just after birth. The condition often runs in families, is three times as common in boys as in girls and often affects children who are ambidextrous (as good with their left hands as they are with their right hands).

Unless dyslexia is recognised early on, children who suffer from it may become withdrawn or difficult at school as they struggle to keep up.

However, once the problem is accurately diagnosed children can be helped by speech therapists, doctors and psychologists. And, of course, by parents who should offer lots of support and love.

EAR ACHE

A narrow tube—the eustachian tube—connects the ear to the nose and if, as a result of a head cold, an infection of the glands or an allergy, this tube becomes blocked, the pressure change which results causes pain inside the ear. This pain can be persistent or intermittent, mild or excruciating and may or may not be accompanied by other signs.

That is the commonest cause of ear ache but there are others. If there is any foreign object inside the ear this can cause pain. So can impacted wax, boils and other localised infections.

Ear ache can also stem from bad teeth, a sore throat or mumps. Cold weather or winds which produce muscle spasm can also cause ear ache.

If ear ache occurs temporarily and briefly after a spell outside in the cold it can usually be ignored. In all other circumstances it must be investigated by a doctor.

In very small children, persistent crying for no obvious reason is often caused by ear ache. If a young child pulls on her ear or rubs it, that should be taken as a sign of ear ache.

If a child who is just getting over a cold wakes up with ear ache and a temperature, the chances are that he or she has developed an infection known as otitis media.

While waiting for medical advice a hot water bottle, wrapped in a thin towel and placed against the ear, will usually give relief. Painkillers such as paracetamol are also useful.

I do not recommend you to use any of the proprietary drops or medicines designed to be put directly into the ear. Under some circumstances (when, for example, the ear drum has ruptured) these can produce complications of their own.

Nor should you try to remove wax or any foreign bodies (such as peas, small toys, sweets or any one of the hundred and one things that children love stuffing into the ears). It's all to easy to push whatever it is you are trying to get out further into the ear, making it even more difficult for an expert to remove it later. It is much safer to ask your doctor to remove the wax or foreign object in the first place.

In the normal, healthy ear sound waves pass down the ear canal to the drum. There they make the drum vibrate; these vibrations are, in turn, transmitted across the middle ear. The vibrations are then passed on to the inner ear where a special organ called the cochlea converts the vibrations into electrical impulses. These impulses are then carried via a special nerve to the brain. The inner ear also contains the semi circular canals which control the sense of balance.

Any disease which affects one or both ears, or which affects the external canal, the bones of the middle ear, the inner ear or the nerve which carries impulses to the brain, can cause deafness. The extent and site of the damage will decide the extent of the deafness.

If the ear ache is caused by something obstructing the

external canal (impacted wax for example) then the blockage will stop sound waves passing down to the drum. This deafness is, of course, temporary. There can also be some deafness accompanying the infection otitis media but this is usually temporary.

Ear ache is not catching in most circumstances; even if it is caused by an ear infection the condition will not be infectious. However, if there is any discharge from the ear this must be regarded as potentially infective.

Sometimes swimming can cause ear ache. The ear's defences seem to be lowered by constant soaking in water. Children with colds shouldn't go swimming since the combination of lowered bodily defences and cold bugs can produce ear ache.

To tell whether the pain of ear ache is inside the ear or in the outer ear you can try tugging gently on the lobe. If the pain comes from an infection deep inside the ear this won't make any difference. If the pain is produced by an infection in the outer ear this will cause additional pain.

When the eustachian tube is blocked it seals off the middle ear. Secretions continue to pour into the space but these are now trapped. If and when they become infected pus will form. This pus will put pressure on the ear drum and so cause pain.

Eventually the pressure may be great enough to rupture the ear drum. When that happens pus, and sometimes some blood too, will flow from the outer ear. Because the ruptured ear drum is no longer under so much pressure the ache may be relieved as the fluid escapes.

It is not a good idea to put cotton wool into the ear to soak up the escaping pus. Let the discharge drain and get well away from the ear as quickly as possible.

A ruptured ear drum will usually heal without any difficulty and with no loss of hearing afterwards. Only when the drum is ruptured repeatedly may hearing loss arise.

It is important to have ear complaints treated as soon as possible to prevent recurrent damage to the drum. Most children who have a lot of ear trouble grow out of it when they reach the age of eight or nine, and their drainage system is more effective.

For pain caused by an infection your doctor will probably prescribe an antibiotic. If the pain and infection are severe and persistent and are caused by great pressure inside the ear, an ear nose and throat specialist may make a small hole in the drum to release the pus.

Children who have had recurrent ear infections sometimes have small plastic tubes inserted into their drums to allow pus to drain out without any pressure, any rupture of the drum or any consequent damage. These small tubes allow air into the middle ear space, and assist drainage down the eustachian tube.

ECZEMA

Skin with eczema (dermatitis) is usually dry, red, itchy and swollen. It can also be blistered, weeping and raw–looking. Any fluid that has leaked from the skin may dry to form a crust. Because the affected area is often itchy it may get infected from scratching.

There are several different types of eczema:

1   Irritant eczema. The skin can be irritated by a huge range of substances. In children and babies it is often saliva and urine. In adults detergents, bleaches and soap powders are common culprits.

2   Allergic contact eczema. The symptoms are often similar to those of irritant eczema and may sometimes develop after repeated contact over months or even years. The allergen producing the reaction can often be identified through patch testing on the skin and the most common are nickel, rubber, sticking plaster and plants.

3   Allergic eczema. Skin rashes of the eczema type can be caused by eating certain foods or by taking drugs which produce an allergic reaction (penicillin and sulphonamide are the two commonest drugs to produce allergic reactions). Almost any food can produce allergic eczema but most often it will be eggs and dairy products.

4   Inherited eczema (also known as atopic eczema) is the commonest type of eczema seen in young children. It

usually develops between the ages of 3 months and 2 years and starts first on the face and nappy area, spreading in later years to the neck, hands, wrists and the fronts of the arms and legs. It can diminish by the age of 5. There is evidence suggesting that this type of eczema is less common in children who have been breast fed: bottle fed babies are seven times more likely to develop the condition.

ELECTRICITY

8 tips to help you avoid the hidden dangers

Electricity is almost certainly more dangerous than you think and could endanger your health. The present state of affairs is like the correlation between smoking and lung cancer 30 years ago. It has been estimated that a third of all childhood cancers are caused by electrical fields.

- Children whose mothers used electric blankets when they were pregnant are two and a half times more likely to develop brain tumours.
- Children who live in houses near power distribution lines are two or three times more likely to die of leukaemia or brain tumours.
- Men who worked alongside electricity power lines were found to be seven times more likely to develop leukaemia.

Here's some simple advice on what can you do to reduce your chances—and the chances of anyone in your family—of being killed by electrical fields:

1　Don't have mains powered radios, answering machines, clocks or other electrical devices unnecessarily close to any member of your family, especially the heads of their beds. Battery operated appliances are probably safer. Don't sleep close to a meter cupboard, even if it's on the other side of a wall.

2　Don't allow your children to sit within two and a half or three feet of the front, sides or back of a Visual Display Terminal, a computer or word processor.

3   If you are pregnant try to keep away from Visual Display Terminals completely. A study of over 1,500 women in California showed that pregnant women who spend more than 20 hours a week working on such terminals have a much greater chance of having a miscarriage.

4   If your child's school is within 150 yards of a major electricity supply line ask the authorities to test the electrical fields in classrooms, playground and sports fields.

5   Don't let children sit closer than six feet from your television set when it is switched on. TV sets produce potentially dangerous electrical fields which are stronger the closer you get.

6   Unplug electrical blankets before you or your children get into bed.

7   Don't allow children to sit or stand close to household appliances such as microwave ovens when they are switched on.

8   Try not to live in a home within 150 yards of a major electricity supply line. I think this is probably particularly important if you have small children or are pregnant.

EMERGENCIES AND ACCIDENTS

Practical advice

1   Dial for emergency help. Ring for an ambulance and then ring for a family doctor. If you are away from home ask a passer by to give you the telephone number of a doctor.

2   Do not move the victim any more than you absolutely have to. It is easy to make injuries worse. Don't move anyone who has a suspected back injury.

3   If the accident is on the road get other drivers to park their cars either side of the accident with hazard lights flashing.

4   Broken bones can be painful and look horrifying. But most people who die unnecessarily do so either because they have lost too much blood or because they are not breathing

properly. Without moving the victim too much, make sure that he is breathing all right and look for signs of heavy bleeding.

5   If the victim is unconscious roll him very gently onto his side. Make sure that his tongue hasn't fallen back (it might block his throat and stop him breathing). Do not give an unconscious patient anything to eat or drink.

6   Keep the victim warm with a rug, jacket, coat or blanket.

7   Try to look calm even if you don't feel calm. Try to offer the victim reassurance. Be firm, calm and reassuring with other passers by. If the victim is conscious talk to him. Find out if there is anyone he would like you to call.

EPILEPSY

4 tips on dealing with a patient who has had an epileptic fit

Epilepsy is not a single disease but a group of disorders which produce convulsions and a loss of consciousness. Epilepsy can start at any age and the fits are produced by a sudden release of electrical energy within the brain. It can be a temporary condition or more or less permanent.

There is often no known cause when epilepsy develops although accidents, wounds and injuries can all cause epilepsy as can excessive heat or disturbances in calcium or sugar metabolism. All these factors cause epilepsy by their effect on the brain.

During an epileptic fit the release of electrical energy within the brain interferes with muscles in many different ways. The nature of the symptoms will depend on the site and size of the electrical disturbance.

The most common and most dramatic type of epileptic fit is known as a grand mal attack or seizure. The patient will suddenly go unconscious, his limbs and trunk will stiffen and then there will be a general flailing and jerking of the muscles. A major fit can be very alarming for onlookers, particularly if they haven't seen one before.

Immediately before a grand mal attack sufferers will often get a strange warning sensation. They'll feel that something is about to happen and they'll sometimes cry out. This warning sensation is known as the aura.

The other type of epileptic fit is known as the petit mal seizure. In this type of fit the patient may simply lose consciousness for a few seconds. He may appear to daydream or his attention may wander. There isn't a lot of movement but there may be some fluttering of the eyelids or nodding of the head.

Here are some guidelines on what should you do if someone has an epileptic fit:

1 Turn the patient onto his side so that he will not swallow saliva or any food he may vomit.

2 Don't try to hold him down. Don't try to put anything in his mouth or between his teeth. Don't give anything to eat or drink. Move as much furniture out of the way as possible.

3 Loosen any tight clothing. Undo zips and buttons where possible.

4 Stay with the patient until he has regained full consciousness. They may be confused and will often complain of being sleepy.

☞ *See also* Convulsions and fits.

EXERCISE

10 ways in which exercise can make you healthier, and 6 rules for exercising sensibly

Unless you exercise regularly your health will be at risk and you will be more prone to disorders as varied as arthritis, osteoporosis, heart disease and depression.

Most of us live fairly sedentary lives. We travel in motor cars, buses and trains and we use gadgets and machines to help us cut down the workload in the house and garden. Just count the number of hours you spend sitting down each day!

In a few thousand years' time we may well have adapted to our sedentary existence, but for now our bodies still need exercise.

Many of the diseases which are commonest today are partly caused by the fact that most of us do not exercise enough.

Here's a list of just some of the diseases that can be made *worse* by not doing any exercise and can be made *better* by a well thought out exercise programme.

1   Arthritis: your joints need to keep moving or else they'll seize up.

2   Backache: sitting or standing in one position for long periods can result in strains that can cause long term back trouble.

3   Headaches: without exercise tension builds up in your muscles and pains develop in the head and neck.

4   Anxiety: exercise is one of the best ways of getting rid of stress and tension that will otherwise build up.

5   Circulation problems: without exercise the blood will stagnate in your veins and you will be more likely to suffer from cold hands, cold feet and varicose veins.

6   Depression: regular exercise can help you avoid or fight depression.

7   Heart trouble: without exercise your heart will become weak and flabby – and the slightest exertion will put it under strain. A well thought out exercise programme will improve the power and strength of your heart.

8   Digestive upsets: indigestion, irritable bowel syndrome and many other digestive problems can be made worse by sitting around too much.

9   Obesity: your weight is a result of the amount of food you eat and the amount you burn up through exercise. The more exercise you do the more food you'll burn up – and the slimmer you'll get. More important still, if you exercise regularly your muscle tone will improve and you'll *look* slimmer and healthier.

10 Sleeplessness: regular exercise will help you sleep better without pills.

So, how much exercise should you take and what should you do?

The first thing you must do is check with your doctor before you undertake an exercise programme.

Then try to find a gym with a good coach, a well run aerobics class or a sports club that you can join.

A good coach is vital: he or she will show you how to take your pulse before and after every exercise session. Within a few weeks you should notice that your pulse will go back to its normal rate quicker and quicker after exercising. You should also notice that your normal pulse rate gets lower as you get fitter. One of the by–products of taking up an exercise programme is that you'll meet new friends with whom you can share the trials and tribulations of getting fit. You'll do better and get more out of your exercise programme if it is *fun*, so try to choose a type of exercise that you think you'll enjoy.

Whatever you choose you should try to combine three separate elements:

- aerobic exercise to improve your heart and general fitness;
- weight training to improve your muscle strength and bone density;
- stretching to improve your suppleness and flexibility.

Allocate time for exercise and stick to it. If you decide to exercise only when you've got a free moment you'll never do anything. You need to set aside time for a properly organised exercise programme. But it need not be much. Three sessions a week will be plenty. You should allow a full hour for each session though to start with you probably won't be able to manage that much. If you are really pushed for time you can squeeze a useful exercise programme into just three twenty minute sessions. Can there be anyone who is so busy that they can't manage one hour a week?

Try to make your exercise time inviolable and give it priority over other, less vital tasks.

You don't need a lot of money to take up exercise but do buy the right gear—the best you can afford. Remember: you're not trying to *look* fashionable but you do need shoes that are comfortable and give good support and since you'll be sweating a lot when you start exercising properly you'll need clothes that can be washed often, quickly and easily. Most women—particularly if they are well endowed—find a special support bra a boon.

Finally, remember the most important rule for exercise: it should never hurt. Pain is your body's way of saying *stop*. If you ignore a pain—and attempt to blunder bravely through the pain barrier—you will almost certainly injure yourself.

Rules for exercise

In order to make sure that you build up your physical endurance levels slowly and carefully—and without injury—you should follow these simple rules:

Rule 1

Always talk to your doctor first—and get his approval and permission for your planned exercise programme.

Rule 2

It is vitally important that before an exercise session you should make sure you loosen your joints and warm up your muscles as well as you can. If you exercise with cold muscles and stiff joints you will increase your chances of acquiring an injury. Similarly, it is important that you cool down after an exercise session. A good aerobics teacher will always make sure that her or his class members all warm up and cool down properly.

Rule 3

If you exercise every day you will become mentally and physically tired. So try to take a rest day between exercise sessions. To get the best result from your exercise programme try to exercise three times a week. (If you are to benefit properly you should exercise at least twice a week and no more than five times a week).

Rule 4

You should be slightly out of breath and sweating a little by the middle of a good exercise session.

Rule 5

If you are going to benefit fully, an exercise session should last at least twenty minutes. Do not exercise for too long until you

have attained a reasonable standard of fitness.
Rule 6
Always talk to a good coach before you start exercising. Get him or her to help you with advice. And make sure that he or she knows about any illness or medical condition you may have.

FADDY EATING

Does it matter?

Over half a century ago an American doctor organised a piece of medical research which produced some astonishing results about children's eating habits. The research was subsequently verified by other workers but was never really given the publicity or the acclaim it deserved.

The purpose of the study was to find out what happens when small children between six months and four and a half years old are allowed to select their own food without any guidance from parents, dieticians or other adults.

Amazingly, the results showed very clearly that even quite young children are perfectly capable of managing their own diets if they are given the right amount of freedom and the opportunity to choose what they eat, how much they eat and when they eat it.

Children (like adults) have in-built appetite control centres capable of regulating their food intake with remarkable precision. They will eat the right mix of protein, fat and carbohydrate. They will automatically take all the necessary vitamins and minerals. And they will even choose a diet designed to avoid the development of constipation and diarrhoea.

There is, of course, one very important rider to all this. And that is that if you are going to allow your child to take over responsibility for his own eating habits then you must consider his eating habits on a long term basis—that is, you have got to give him time to adjust and to experiment a little with his diet.

If he doesn't ever eat an unbalanced diet then his appetite control centre will never be stretched and he will never learn. And just as a diabetic will only ever really get to grips with his

disorder when he has been low on sugar and has had a hypo-
glycaemic attack, so your child will only be able to recognise
the nudges and pressures from his appetite control centre when
he has eaten too much of something and not enough of something else.

None of this is easy.

Many mothers will be quite unable to sit back and relax
while their four year olds starve for twelve hours and then eat
two bags of crisps and twelve jelly sandwiches. And I don't seriously suggest that any mother should even try to do anything
as extreme as allow her child so much freedom.

But what mothers can learn from this is that it is wise to relax
a little about your child's eating habits. There is no need to turn
the kitchen and the dining room into a battle zone. Battling
with your child over what he eats, when he eats it and how
much he eats will wear you out and make your child all the
more determined to have his own way.

The message is simple: don't push too hard. Let your child
have some freedom. Allow him to make some of the decisions
for himself about what he wants to eat. The chances are that his
body knows better than you do what he needs. The appetite
control centre which decides what your child needs also hands
out information about the amount of food your child needs. If
you try to force your child to eat what you think he should eat,
when you think he should eat and in the quantities you think
he should eat then you will batter his appetite control centre
into insensitivity.

If your child is not hungry don't be too upset about him
missing an odd meal. If he doesn't want to finish all his sprouts
then relax—just give him less next time.

If you give him some freedom then he will grow up with an
appetite control centre in working order and a waistline which
is likely to stay permanently trim.

FAINTING

Fainting is a temporary loss of consciousness caused by a reduction in the flow of blood to the brain—something which is outside voluntary control.

Someone who is about to faint may complain of feeling light headed or nauseous. He will probably be pale and clammy and have a glazed look in his eyes.

The individual who faints will fall down into a horizontal position, making the blood supply to the brain much easier to restore. That's what happens from a physiological point of view but the causes are not so straightforward.

Fainting can be caused by a hot and stuffy atmosphere, by low blood sugar levels or a sudden change of position.

Another major cause is anxiety—there is no doubt that this is often the factor behind the mass fainting sessions which occur at large gatherings.

The only risk is usually one of injury caused by the actual process of fainting to the ground. Consciousness will return as soon as the blood supply to the brain is restored.

Anyone who has just recovered from fainting should not stand up too quickly. Gently bring him into a sitting position with his legs bent and then place the head between the knees. Call your doctor to check out a cause for the fainting attack.

FEET

10 ways to look after your child's feet

Most children start life with wonderful feet. But carelessness and thoughtlessness can eventually lead to serious problems such as bunions, callouses, corns and worse. Many people with bad feet develop serious back problems as the years go by. Because they cannot walk properly their joints—and their spines—suffer terribly.

Here are ten simple rules that will help you keep your child's feet healthy:

1   Feet get bigger as the day goes on. It is always a good idea to buy new shoes after lunch. There is a real risk that if you buy new shoes in the morning they will 'pinch' when the child wears them in the afternoon. When your child is

being measured for new shoes he should stand and both feet should be measured. Not many people have two feet of identical size and although shops won't usually want to split a pair of shoes you should make sure that you buy a pair big enough for your child's bigger foot. Make sure that he tries on both shoes. To check that a shoe is big enough see if you can push your finger between your child's heel and the back of the shoe. If you can't then the chances are that the shoes are going to be too tight.

2   Trainers, pumps and plimsolls may be fashionable and may seem comfortable but they are not suitable for everyday use. Often the material is such that the feet cannot breathe properly—so they sweat far more than is good for them. And since not all pumps are available in half sizes it is not always possible to get a good fit. It is worth remembering that rubber or synthetic shoes tend to make the feet sweat. Shoes that have laces or adjustable straps are better for the feet than shoes that don't—especially if your child has a high instep.

3   Don't be in too much of a rush to put a baby into shoes. Babies really do not need to wear shoes until they are walking by themselves. Until they are walking they are better off barefoot. Tiny shoes may look rather sweet but they can cramp a growing foot.

4   Make sure that baby growers, romper suits and stretch suits are big enough. If they aren't then your baby's feet will get compressed just as badly as they would in ill fitting shoes.

5   Tight socks are bad for children. It is as important to make sure that socks are big enough as it is to make sure that shoes are big enough. Make sure that your child changes his shoes or stockings every day to keep his feet in good condition.

6   Make sure that your children always wash and dry their feet carefully and thoroughly. It is the failure to dry the feet properly (for example, after showering following a visit to the gym) that can lead to all sorts of foot infections. Drying in between the toes is vitally important. Many teenagers spend hours worrying about their faces but no time at all

looking after their feet.

7 Don't buy Sunday best shoes for children. If you do then the chances are that your child will be wearing his 'best' shoes long after he has grown out of them. It is much better to buy just one pair of shoes and let the child wear them all the time.

8 If your child has dry skin on his feet use a moisturising cream to protect them.

9 Remember that high heeled shoes and shoes with pointed toes may be all right for parties or occasional special wear but they are really not suitable for everyday use. Shoes that are worn every day—particularly for walking or standing—need to be comfortable and well fitting. Millions of women have terrible feet—and suffer from leg and back problems—because when they were teenagers they insisted on wearing fashionable shoes. High heeled shoes force the feet into a terrible and quite unnatural position and tend to cram the toes into the front of the shoes. It is hardly surprising that after wearing such shoes for a few years many women have feet that look terrible and that make any sort of walking a torturous experience.

10 Teach your child how to look after his toe nails. He should not cut them too close at the edges—otherwise he risks getting ingrowing toe nails, which can be difficult and painful to treat. Toe nails should be cut straight across the top.

Foot problems

Two our of every five people have foot problems. Among older people problems are even commoner—with four out of every five having something significantly wrong with their feet.

Because foot problems are rarely dangerous or life threatening they are often not taken seriously. Doctors don't rush around in hospitals to tackle bunions or ingrowing toe nails. But, apart from the fact that they are often inconvenient and painful, foot problems contribute to serious disorders. Back and joint troubles in adulthood, for example, are often caused by or made worse by food disorders which started in childhood.

Here are some of the commonest problems likely to affect your feet:

ATHLETE'S FOOT

In this condition the skin between and under the toes is damp, itchy and inflamed. It may look white or red. Nylon socks tend to make athlete's foot worse as do plastic shoes or pumps which do not allow the feet to breathe. You can buy anti fungal creams from a pharmacy to help deal with this condition. To prevent athlete's foot wear cotton or woollen socks to reduce the amount of sweating and dry your feet thoroughly.

BUNIONS

Badly fitting shoes—often with high heels and pointed toes—can cause bunions. The toes are forced out of position by tight shoes with the result that a bony lump appears at the side of the foot. The only way to deal with a bunion permanently is to see a surgeon!

CALLUSES

These are caused by wearing shoes that are too big or too small, by constantly wearing high heeled shoes or simply by being too fat. Calluses are patches of hard skin produced by pressure. Losing weight may help. Rubbing on a moisturising cream will help though you can also get rid of hard patches of skin by gently, regularly rubbing with a pumice stone (obtainable from the pharmacy). To avoid the problem make sure that you wear well fitting shoes and socks, tights or stockings.

CORNS

Tightly or badly fitting shoes cause corns—which can be very painful. The skin becomes very hard and thick and may press on underlying nerves. You need to see a chiropodist to get a corn removed.

INGROWING TOE NAILS

Toe nails grow into the skin when they are not cut properly. You should always cut toe nails straight across to avoid this problem developing. Ingrowing toe nails are very painful. Sometimes a chiropodist can help but often surgery is needed.

WARTS

Warts on the feet are known as verrucae. They are caused by a virus. You can buy remedies from a pharmacist. Or see a chiropodist. Verrucae are infectious. Verrucae are often caught in swimming baths and changing rooms.

Remember: see your doctor or a chiropodist at the first sign of any foot problem. If you leave a problem in the hope that it will go away, the chances are that it will get worse.

☞ *See also* Flat feet.

FEVER

5 tips for coping

The normal temperature within the human body is 98.6 degrees Fahrenheit (37 degrees centigrade). When the temperature rises above this the patient is said to have a fever. A fever is not an illness—it is a symptom.

When the body temperature rises in response to an internal infection the high temperature may help speed recovery by killing the bugs causing the infection. It is only if a fever rises too high or too quickly that it poses serious problems.

The traditional way to tell whether or not someone has a high temperature is to place the back of your hand on the patient's forehead. But hands can give misleading results and the thermometer gives a far better result. It really isn't as difficult to use as many people think. And these days battery operated electronic thermometers are available which provide a digital readout—so you don't have to struggle to find the level of a thin column of mercury.

Although the normal body temperature is 98.6 degrees Fahrenheit, in practice it will often vary by a degree or two at different times of the day. The body's temperature is usually at its highest in the late afternoon and at its lowest at about 4 am. Temperature can also rise as a result of exercise.

The rate at which a fever rises is important—particularly in children when a fast rising temperature can lead to a febrile convulsion. If a patient's temperature is rising fast try to reduce the rate at which it rises by sponging with tepid (not cold) water, by taking the patient's clothes off and by opening a window—while waiting for medical help to arrive.

Tips for coping with a fever (*after* calling for the doctor):

1 Do not make the mistake of wrapping up a patient who is hot. If you do that you will simply send his temperature soaring even higher. The patient who is hot will, by and large, need fewer clothes, not more.

2 Sponging with tepid or even warm water will help to reduce the temperature. Do not use cold water because if you do you will reduce the superficial blood circulation and send the temperature up instead of down. You don't need to tepid sponge unless the temperature is above 102 degrees Fahrenheit or is rising rapidly.

3 If the patient's temperature is 102 degrees Fahrenheit or more and he appears unwell then you may be able to bring down his temperature by using soluble aspirin or paracetamol. But you should only give these or any other medicines under the supervision of a doctor.

4 To avoid dehydration make sure that your patient takes plenty of fluid. Food doesn't matter as much as fluid.

5 If your patient wants to stay in bed then let him. But if he wants to get up then you should let him unless the doctor has said 'no' to this.

FLAT FEET

We all have flat feet when we are born. Arches only develop on the inner edges of our feet as we get older. As the muscles of our feet and legs develop so these arches get stronger.

Proper foot arches don't usually develop until a child reaches the age of 4 or 5. Before that flat feet are normal.

To find out whether your child's feet are flat get him to stand on tip toes. You should be able to see an arch developing. Alternatively, get him to dip his foot in water and then check out the imprint his foot makes.

To help feet develop properly encourage children to walk about in bare feet indoors. And make sure that shoes don't cramp or pinch the feet.

One in twenty children will grow up with flat feet. You can help your child develop an arch by encouraging him to stand on tip toes regularly. Your doctor may suggest that the shoe shop adds an inner raise to help arches develop. Or, if necessary, he will fix an appointment with an orthopaedic surgeon (though that isn't usually necessary).

FOOD

Eating healthily

It is often said that you are what you eat—and it's true!

Your body's cells are constantly dying and being replaced. As the years go by organs and tissues are for ever being rebuilt. The raw materials for this constant renovation project are the foods you eat. So, clearly, the better your diet the healthier you will be.

Recent research has proved that your chances of suffering from one of the big killer diseases—cancer, heart disease, strokes and so on—are largely dependent on your eating habits. Eat the wrong foods and you will dramatically reduce your chances of living a long and healthy life.

With the possible exception of being born to healthy parents (and there isn't much you can do about that once you've been born!) eating a well balanced and healthy diet is the most important thing you can do.

So, what *is* a healthy diet? The answer is simpler than you might think.

The first thing you must remember is that you mustn't eat too much. Most of us stuff ourselves with food—and make ourselves ill.

Try to get into the habit of eating when you are hungry and

stopping eating when you are full (or, better still, just before you feel full!). Don't eat just because everyone else is eating. Don't nibble because you are bored or miserable. And don't leave the table wishing you hadn't eaten so much.

Next, try to remember that a balanced diet is vital. There aren't many foods that will kill you in small quantities. But all foods will kill you if you eat too much of them. One biscuit won't kill you. But living on nothing but biscuits won't do you much good.

Small, regular meals are probably better for you than huge, irregular meals.

Just remember that your body has to rebuild cells out of what you eat! Next time you're stuffing yourself with chips or ice cream ask yourself how your body is going to make red blood cells out of what you're eating.

If you eat meat, try to cut down on animal fats. Too much fatty food will increase your chances of developing cancer and heart disease. Eat low fat margarine instead of butter and avoid red meat as much as possible. Eat no more than three eggs a week.

And try to eat plenty of fresh vegetables. (But don't overcook them because if you do you'll destroy much of the goodness in them.) Eat plenty of fresh fruit too. Apples, bananas and oranges are all good for you.

To increase your fibre intake eat wholemeal bread and brown rice. And cut down your consumption of sugar because too much sugar is a common cause of obesity and tooth decay.

FRACTURES

A simple fracture is one in which the bones have not broken through the skin.

A compound or open fracture is one in which the bones have broken through the skin—therefore increasing the chance of infection.

A comminuted fracture is one in which the bone is broken in several places.

A displaced fracture is one in which the two ends of broken bone are not in contact with one another and may need to be realigned before the bone can be set again.

An undisplaced fracture is one in which the two ends of broken bone are still in contact with one another.

An impacted fracture is one in which the two ends of broken bone are pushed into each other like two cars fixed together after an accident.

A complicated fracture is one in which the broken bone has damaged a nerve or blood vessel.

All fractures, or suspected fractures, need emergency medical help.

GALL BLADDER—AND GALL STONES

The gall bladder is a small bag (the size of a tiny purse) where bile is stored. Bile is a mixture of acids, pigments and cholesterol which help to absorb fats. Your gall bladder is tucked away under your liver (and under your rib cage) on your right hand side.

You can manage without your gall bladder. If the gall bladder is removed bile flows directly into your intestines. The gall bladder is just a warehouse.

The most likely problem with a gall bladder is that you'll develop gall stones. These are usually made of cholesterol. But they can be made of calcium or pigment.

Gall stones do not always mean trouble. Literally millions of people have gall stones without knowing that they are there. Problems usually only develop when the stones get stuck moving out of the gall bladder. They are often found on routine X-rays.

Gall stones should probably only be removed when they cause trouble. Surgeons used to take out all gall bladders when they'd found stones. These days most doctors agree that gall stones that don't cause any symptoms can be left where they are. One survey showed that as many people die having their gall bladders removed as are killed by gall bladder stones. So the operation should only be done when it's really necessary (e.g. when the stones are causing pain).

The traditional operation is quite simple and relatively safe. The surgeon makes a cut in the abdominal wall, reaches in and cuts out the gall bladder. Patients stay in hospital for a week or so and need up to six weeks sick leave.

Some surgeons are now using lasers to cut out the gall bladder. They then suck out the bladder and stones through a tiny tube. This operation—through a keyhole sized scar—involves a hospital stay of no more than one or two days. And patients can be back at work within two weeks. But this operation does need a specially trained surgeon.

Some surgeons are using a technique called lithotripsy—which shatters the gallstones. And some doctors are now prescribing drugs which dissolve gall stones. There seems a good chance that within a few years time doctors will be able to remove gall stones without an operation at all.

GERMAN MEASLES

See Rubella.

GLANDULAR FEVER

Also known as infectious mononucleosis, this is a viral infection in which the initial symptoms usually include a high temperature, headache, sore throat and swollen lymph glands.

Glandular fever usually affects young people and because it is commonly transmitted by kissing it is sometimes known as the 'kissing disease'. A blood test can be done to confirm the diagnosis.

The majority of patients make a good recovery after four to six weeks. Drug therapy is not usually needed. Patients often feel depressed, tired and sleepy for several months afterwards.

GOUT

Any joint in the body can be affected by gout but the big toes are the joints most commonly involved. The ankles, knees, wrists, elbows and fingers are also common sites for gout. The disease usually affects men rather than women (in a ratio of 20 to 1), is particularly common among individuals between the ages of 35 and 60, and runs in families.

Most gout sufferers are rather overweight and often also have high blood pressure.

Gout develops when the levels of uric acid in the blood get too high and uric acid crystals accumulate in the joints, where they may eventually damage the joint surfaces and the bones— producing long term symptoms rather similar to those associated with osteoarthritis.

Normally, uric acid is formed when waste products are broken down in the body. In a healthy individual the uric acid is excreted in the urine but gout sufferers fail to get rid of all the uric acid their bodies are making. There are several possible reasons for this. The kidneys may be damaged, and not getting rid of uric acid properly. There may be an inherited tendency to high levels of uric acid. Or the problem may simply be caused by eating too many foods which are broken down to produce high levels of uric acid. Prescribed drugs can sometimes trigger a high uric acid level—and an attack of gout.

Gout usually begins with a fairly sudden onset of severe pain in a joint which is usually swollen and rather bluish red in colour. There may also be a moderate fever. The symptoms of gout tend to come and go quite unexpectedly. The first attack usually begins with an itchy, swollen toe which gradually becomes painful. Treatment of gout is important because if uric acid levels are allowed to remain high, the kidneys may be damaged by an accumulation of crystals.

Gout is fairly common. But many sufferers only get one or two attacks a year.

Patients with acute gout are usually advised to rest. Anti-inflammatory drugs are sometimes prescribed to ease pain and some patients need long term treatment with drugs which prevent the accumulation of uric acid or which help the kidneys to get rid of uric acid and thereby help prevent pain recurring.

Many patients notice an improvement in their condition if they lose weight and avoid certain foods or drugs. Foods which are particularly likely to cause problems include: meat extracts, game, asparagus, spinach, strawberries, rhubarb, fish roe, herring, salmon, whitebait, liver, kidneys and sweetbreads. Drinks which can cause gout include: carbonated drinks, beer, sparkling wines, port, champagne and many other kinds of alcohol.

GUM DISEASE

Gum disease is one of the commonest of all diseases but it can be beaten. Gum and tooth disease are inextricably linked—indeed gum disease is responsible for the loss of millions of teeth. Your dentist will probably be able to help by cleaning your teeth properly but if you're going to conquer the problem permanently you have to start taking more care of your mouth.

Check out your toothbrush. If the bristles don't spring back into action when you press down on them you need a replacement. Buy one with a small head (so that you can get into difficult places) and avoid very hard bristles (which will make the bleeding worse).

When you clean your teeth clean your gums too. Ask for an appointment with your dentist's hygienist (most good practices have one these days) and she'll check out your tooth cleaning regime. One really good clean twice a day is better than a perfunctory rub four times a day. Try to make sure each tooth is cleaned.

And use dental floss to remove food debris from between your teeth—that will help your gums too.

HAEMORRHOIDS

Haemorrhoids (also known as piles) are varicose veins around the anus. They are very common during pregnancy and after childbirth. Some people are just prone to them. The symptoms include rectal bleeding, and pain when the bowels are opened. Itching and a mucous discharge may also occur. Eating a high fibre diet and drinking plenty of fluids may help patients with modest piles. More serious sufferers may need surgery of one sort or another.

HAIR PROBLEMS

Dry hair, greasy hair, hair loss, excess hair

Dry hair

Dry hair is brittle, coarse and difficult to comb or set. It also breaks easily and splits at the ends. If you have dry hair there are several things worth remembering:

1 Heat makes dry hair worse.
2 Frequent brushing may help by stimulating the production of natural oils.
3 Wash your hair less frequently.
4 Ignore people who tell you to eat an oil–rich diet. It won't help.
5 Use a conditioner
6 Try rubbing a little olive oil onto your hair half an hour before washing it.
7 Avoid perming or colouring the hair if possible.

Greasy hair

It is the sebum—a fatty secretion produced by glands on the scalp—which makes hair greasy and if these glands are irritated in any way they increase their production of sebum. So, if you are prone to greasy hair don't wear a style which needs brushing or combing too much.

If you wash greasy hair too often you will simply make the condition worse so you need to compromise and wash it every two or three days. Don't use very hot water and don't scrub your scalp too much.

When buying shampoos look for one that is free of additives and avoid combined conditioners which may add to the grease problem.

Hair loss

Loss of hair most commonly affects men. Male pattern baldness is inherited and there is no cure. Stress is the next commonest cause and affects both men and women—though hair often grows back again afterwards. Some drugs—particularly those used to treat cancer—can cause hair loss.

Excess hair

Body hair is not considered acceptable by many women and some will go to extraordinary lengths to remove it. Apart from specific medical remedies there are six main ways to get rid of unwanted hair:

1   Cutting it off—usually in the form of shaving with a razor. This will not make the re-growth coarser but it will feel stubbly to begin with.

2   Chemical removal usually using a depilatory cream. These can produce a variety of unpleasant allergy reactions so must be tested first on a small patch of skin.

3   Waxing—warm wax is applied to the skin, allowed to set and then pulled off taking the hairs with it. Best done by a professional.

4   Plucking—removing hairs by pulling them out with tweezers. Always remove in the direction of the hair growth. Don't remove single hairs that are associated with a mole until you've checked with a doctor.

5   Electrolysis—a more permanent method of removal using an electrical impulse. Should only be performed by a professional.

6   Sugaring—when a paste of sugar is rolled over the skin, trapping and removing the hairs.

HANGNAILS

'Hangnails' – little bits of nail splitting off along the sides of the nails—are unsightly as well as being a nuisance. Occasionally, if you catch them in a jumper or towel, they can be very painful. Although hangnails are very common there isn't any magical remedy, so don't bother buying anything special from the beauty counter and don't try pulling off the slivers of skin which you might find sticking up by the side of the nail. Instead, cut them off neatly with a pair of sharp nail scissors.

Apart from a few which are caused by careless manicuring most hangnails probably develop through too much hand washing and not enough drying.

Washing dishes, clothes, food and children means that the average woman's nails are soaked over a dozen times a day. Usually they're dried perfunctorily on a damp scrap of bald towel. And nails don't just get dipped in water! They spend hours soaked in powerful detergents and washing powders. It's hardly surprising that nails get weakened and cracked.

The simplest way to avoid nail damage is to wear rubber gloves—preferably with cotton liners. Alternatively keep a pot of barrier cream next to the kitchen sink and use it.

And remember: when your hands have been wet, rinse them thoroughly and dry them carefully.

HANGOVERS

Contrary to popular opinion, hangovers are not an inevitable consequence of drinking too much. Hangovers are entirely optional and are quite easily avoided (unless you're a masochist and enjoy waking up with your tongue pasted to the roof of your mouth, eyeballs foggy on the inside and such an acutely enhanced sense of hearing that you're likely to wince at the noise made by a falling sock).

There is one big problem with the world's only really effective hangover cure. For it to work properly you have to act before you go to bed.

The evil symptoms of a hangover, the throbbing skull, the dry mouth and other horrors too awful to mention, are largely inspired by the fact that alcohol is a diuretic: it makes your body get rid of water. So when you wake up regretting the night before you are suffering because your entire body is dehydrated.

Although it is the major cause of morning distress, alcohol induced dehydration is not quite the only cause of the symptoms that bedevil the morning after a good night before. Mixing your drinks can also make life miserable. Brandy, champagne and red wine are particularly poor mixers. Stick to one type of alcohol and you'll benefit enormously.

The only truly effective way to beat a hangover is to make sure that you drink enough plain fluid to counteract the dehydrating effect of the alcohol you're consuming. And you have to do this as you go along or, at the latest, just before you fall into bed. By the following morning it will be far, far too late. Just slip into the kitchen every hour or so and knock back a tumbler full of water. A couple of pints of plain water spread through the evening should do the trick.

(Though, of course, I have to point out that avoiding excessive drinking is a much healthier way of avoiding a hangover!)

HAY FEVER

3 tips for coping

People who don't get it always think of it as a bit of a joke; at worst a mild inconvenience.

But the growing millions of hay fever sufferers know that it is anything but a joke. It can turn summer every year into a nightmare; it can ruin examination hopes; disrupt work; wreck sporting careers and prove irritating and embarrassing almost beyond belief. And although hay fever itself isn't usually life threatening it can—and often does—trigger potentially serious asthma attacks.

Hay fever is caused by an allergy to pollen.

In just the same way that some people break out in a rash if they eat strawberries or take penicillin tablets and others are allergic to cheap jewellery or certain types of detergent, so hay fever sufferers are allergic to pollen. And because the pollen is floating around in the air it is the most sensitive parts of our bodies—our eyes and nasal membranes especially—which suffer most.

In the spring it's pollen from trees such as plane, elm, hazel, birch, oak and alder which cause the trouble. And in the summer months—when most victims suffer— it's pollen from grasses and weeds that trigger the sneezing and the watery, itchy eyes that are the most common symptoms.

One of the most surprising things about hay fever is that it has been gradually getting commoner for over a century.

And that puzzles some experts because many trees have been chopped down or blown down and these days farmers frequently cut grass before it flowers to make silage for winter animal feed. Theoretically all this should reduce the amount of pollen—and the incidence of hay fever.

Top international experts explain the increase in the number of hay fever sufferers in three ways:

● Car exhaust fumes are the most likely explanation. Doctors used to tell hay fever sufferers to keep away from the country. These days the advice has changed and doctors tell patients to avoid towns and cities where traffic is heavy and the air is polluted. The more polluted the air is the more vulnerable our bodies become to pollen.

● Hay fever isn't contagious but it is passed on in families. One of your ancestors could have passed the allergy on to you and dozens of your relatives.

● Living and working in air conditioned, double glazed, centrally heated buildings has made us all more vulnerable to outside hazards such as pollen.

Most sufferers get their first symptoms in their teens or early twenties but hay fever can affect people in their 70s or even 80s. Men seem to suffer more than women. No one is immune. And just because you haven't had it before doesn't mean that you won't get it this summer. Or next.

If you suddenly find yourself complaining of a persistent

runny nose that feels for ever clogged; lots of sneezing; watery, sore, itchy eyes; an itchy, irritated throat and dark circles under your eyes (caused by restricted blood flow near your sinuses) then you could have become a hay fever sufferer.

One bright spot: for most sufferers the worst symptoms seem to become milder or even disappear after fifteen or twenty summers of sneezing.

Amazingly, there is still no cure.

But there are a number of things hay fever sufferers can do to minimise their symptoms.

1   The most effective way to control hay fever symptoms is to take anti–histamine tablets. A few years ago anti–histamines were effective but caused so much drowsiness that most people couldn't take them during the day without falling asleep. These days drug companies have managed to produce effective anti–histamines which produce far less drowsiness. Check with your pharmacist.

2   There are numerous 'alternative' remedies for hay fever. Most are of doubtful value. But many patients claim that homoeopathic remedies work well.

3   Wearing glasses will help protect your eyes from the pollen. The *best* glasses are close fitting, wrap-around 'cycling' sun glasses which are most effective at keeping the pollen at bay. You can get them from cycle or sports shops.

HEADACHE

3 ways of dealing with headaches

Four out of every five people suffer from headaches. Most get their headaches irregularly. Some suffer daily. The headache is the commonest single symptom people complain about.

Unfortunately, doctors don't always treat headaches very well. The main reason for this is that although headaches may be crippling they aren't usually life threatening. Headaches can be excruciatingly painful and can wreck your life in many ways but they won't usually kill you. And doctors have a nasty habit of dismissing problems which make their patients' lives miserable but don't threaten to kill them.

Go and see your doctor with something rare and threatening and you will find yourself surrounded by expensive equipment and men in white coats before you can wince. But turn up with a skull numbing headache and you will probably stagger out two minutes later clutching a prescription for twenty aspirin tablets.

You should, of course, always seek your doctor's advice about a headache—particularly if:

- it follows a head injury
- it is severe, has developed suddenly and without warning
- it is accompanied by a stiff neck
- you also have a temperature
- it lasts for more than 24 hours
- you have recurring headaches
- it develops after you have started medical treatment
- you are worried

But the good news is that most headaches can be tamed because most headaches are caused by stress, pressure and anxiety. Worry about something that has happened can produce a nervous headache—as can worry about something that might happen in the future.

Strains caused by concentrating hard can cause exactly the same symptoms. If you have been crouched over the accounts or hunched over a steering wheel, you are likely to develop a nervous headache.

You can see how the pains develop simply by looking at yourself in the mirror the next time you are worried about something. Look around your eyes—there will be worry lines developing there because you are frowning, squinting and screwing up your eyes. Look at the way your shoulders are hunched.

The nervous tension in your body is producing muscle tension—and the muscle tension is causing your headache.

The headache will probably start in one place and gradually spread over the top of your head. It may be throbbing; it may feel as if you've got a hat on your head that is too tight; it may be a steady, pressing ache. It can last a few minutes to a week or more and may slowly spread to the muscles of your neck and your jaw. Every time you are upset or anxious or unhappy the pain will get worse.

Most people try to deal with headaches of this sort with aspirin or paracetamol. And since both are excellent drugs they will probably work.

But taking a pain killing tablet to cure a nervous headache is rather like pouring water into a car that has a burst radiator hose—it is a *very* short term solution to a potentially long term problem.

Here are a few solutions that do not involve pills.

1   Since muscle tension will be helping to make your headache worse, you can help yourself by deliberately relaxing the muscles of your head and neck.

This is not as difficult as it sounds.

Deliberately clench the muscles of your left hand.

Try it now.

Make the muscles go as tight as you can get them.

Hold your fist in that position while you count up to twenty. You will feel a pain developing.

You can let your fist go loose now.

Much the same sort of thing happens in your head when you are under pressure. The muscles of your face, head and neck all become tight and so you get a pain.

By learning how to relax the muscles around your head you can get rid of a headache.

You need to practise this when you have not got a headache. Screw up your face really tightly. Try to tighten up every muscle in your face. Tense your neck. Get your whole head and neck feeling uncomfortably tight.

Now, slowly, relax all those muscles. Deliberately let them go all loose and floppy. You should be able to feel the tension and the potential pain pour out of them.

Practise this as often as you can. Then, next time you get a nervous headache you will be able to recognise the difference between tensed facial and neck muscles and relaxed face and neck muscles—and you will be able to combat your headache by deliberately letting your muscles go loose.

2   Next time you feel a nervous headache developing try to look at what is happening as objectively as you can.

Try to put everything into perspective.

Often when things go wrong we panic and worry ourselves sick when worrying really isn't going to help at all.

If you are twenty minutes late, sitting frowning in your traffic jam isn't going to help at all. It is just going to mean that when you finally get to your destination you will have a stinking headache and feel absolutely rotten.

Try to think of good things—things that you are looking forward to. Or try to remember good times in the past.

3   Try massaging the muscles of your face and neck with your finger tips. Start at the outside of your eyes. Make little round circular movements with your finger tips. Be slow and gentle. Then gradually work your way down the line of your jaw. Next, massage the bridge of your nose between your thumb and first finger. Then massage your forehead. Finally, use both hands to massage the back of your neck. You will be amazed at how much difference it makes. Move your head forwards and backwards to get rid of some of the tension.

Heart disease

8 tips to protect your heart

Your heart is about the same size as your fist and like every organ in your body it needs a constant supply of oxygen to stay alive. It is remarkably powerful and reliable.

If your heart beats 70 times a minute then it will beat a million and a half times in a year. But you will only notice if the beat becomes irregular in some way.

Blood reaches the muscles of your heart through the two

main coronary arteries—the right and the left. The left divides into two sub branches and if one or both of these main arteries becomes narrowed or blocked then blood won't be able to get through to your heart muscle. Deprived of oxygen the muscle will protest—and you'll collapse in pain.

When someone collapses suddenly from heart disease two things have usually happened.

The first is that the inside of the blood vessel will have slowly been narrowed as fat which has been travelling in the blood stream has stuck to the wall. This is similar to the way in which water pipes can fur up. In many patients who have heart attacks the width of the blood vessel may have been reduced by half.

This slow reduction in the width of the vessel may cause slight chest pains to develop on exercise—these are called anginal pains. But blood vessels can be narrowed by up to 50% without any pain developing.

The second thing that happens to trigger off a sudden heart attack is that a lump of debris that may have broken off the inside of the artery wall somewhere else will get stuck inside the coronary artery—suddenly blocking it completely.

The chances of your heart having narrowed arteries depends very much on your family history. The rate at which your blood vessels 'fur up' depends upon the amount of cholesterol in your blood. And although that is influenced by the amount of fatty food you eat, a tendency to have a high blood cholesterol level can be inherited. There is even a chance that the way you were fed as a baby may affect your chances of having a heart attack. If you were not weaned off the breast or bottle before one year the chances are that you will have a higher blood cholesterol level. If your mother, father or grandparents suffered from heart disease, there is a risk that you too will have a susceptibility to heart trouble.

How to avoid a heart attack

Heart attack victims are getting younger and younger. A third of the men who die suddenly with heart trouble are of working age. An increasing number are still in their thirties. However, most heart attacks can be prevented.

1 Watch what you eat

It has been known for thirty years that there is a link between fatty food and heart disease. Too much fat will clog up your arteries and make your heart work harder. Use a low fat spread instead of butter. Drink skimmed or semi skimmed milk. Limit your consumption of red meat and cut the fat off meat. Eat no more than 2 or 3 eggs a week. In countries where people eat little fat, death rates from heart disease are much lower than in countries where fat consumption is high. Eat *more* high fibre foods such as oat bran, *more* vegetables, *more* beans, *more* garlic and onions and *more* yoghurt.

2 Don't smoke

Poisons in tobacco narrow blood vessels, increase the risk of blood clotting, stop heart muscles working properly and reduce the oxygen flow to your heart. Smoking causes one in four cases of heart disease. Try to give up smoking altogether. If you can't give up cut down or switch to a low tar brand. If you live or work with someone who smokes try to persuade them to give up. Inhaling secondhand smoke can be bad for you too!

2 Lose excess weight

Every extra pound of fat you carry around with you means that your heart has to work harder. If you are more than 14 pounds overweight, you are very much at risk. Try carrying seven 2 lb bags of sugar around with you for an hour to see just how much extra work that extra weight makes your body do. If you've got a roll of fat more than two inches thick anywhere on your body, you need to lose weight *now*. Eat only when you are hungry—and stop eating when you are full.

3 Reduce the amount of coffee you drink

Too much strong coffee or tea can make your heart work harder than it need. Coffee contains a drug called caffeine which is a powerful stimulant.

4 EXERCISE REGULARLY

Exercise will help keep your heart healthy by strengthening its muscles. Men and women who exercise regularly are far less likely to suffer from heart disease than men and women who never exercise. But, remember: exercise should always be fun and never be painful. To get the best result, exercise regularly—two or three times a week—and exercise for between 30 and 60 minutes a session. Check with your doctor before starting an exercise programme and then visit a local gym or properly run aerobics class.

5 DRINK ALCOHOL IN MODERATION

If you drink too much alcohol you will put your heart under strain. But a small amount of booze may help your heart! Some doctors believe that a maximum of two (small) glasses of alcohol a day will help keep your circulation in tip top condition.

6 CONTROL YOUR STRESS

When you are under pressure your heart will beat faster and your blood pressure will rise. Both put your heart under pressure. Long periods of stress can do lasting damage to your heart. Try to avoid unnecessary anxieties. Make sure that you take time out to relax at least once a week. And learn *how* to relax properly.

7 LET YOUR EMOTIONS SHOW

If you hold your emotions in you will put your heart under pressure. So don't be afraid to cry when you are sad, to shout when you are angry and to laugh when you're happy. A stiff upper lip can turn you into a stiff corpse.

8 WATCH OUT FOR EARLY WARNING SIGNS OF TROUBLE

Seek help at the first signs of heart trouble. Symptoms to watch out for include: chest pains, breathlessness, palpitations and a thumping heart—often brought on by stress or sudden, unaccustomed exercise. See your doctor straight away if you notice any of these.

HEREDITARY HEALTH PROBLEMS

Few things affect your health as much as your family history. Good health runs in families. So does poor health. Many of the commonest and most important diseases can be inherited.

But the news isn't all bad.

If you know *which* diseases run in your family you can do things to protect yourself.

First, find out what (if any) diseases your close relatives (parents, grandparents, brothers and sisters) have suffered from. Then check them out on this list and take action to minimise your chances of suffering from the same problem. (This list is not complete and these are by no means the only disorders which can be inherited).

Cancer

If several members of your family have suffered from the same type of cancer (e.g. breast cancer, bowel cancer) inform your doctor and ask for regular checkups.

Diabetes

If you have a family history watch out for early symptoms (excessive thirst, frequent passing of urine, weight loss, boils). Don't get overweight. Limit your sugar intake. Have your urine tested for sugar regularly.

Heart disease

Early symptoms include breathlessness and chest pain. Minimise your risk by staying slim, taking regular exercise and avoiding unnecessary stress. Keep your consumption of fats to a minimum. Don't smoke. Have your blood cholesterol level and blood pressure checked regularly.

Glaucoma

Early symptoms include visual problems and pains in the eye. Have an annual eye test—it will help spot the disease early on. And make sure that your doctor and optician know about the family history.

Ulcers

Indigestion, gastritis and nausea are all early symptoms which warn that an ulcer may be developing. Eat regularly. Avoid foods that upset you. Keep drinking and smoking to an absolute minimum. Learn to control your stress.

HERPES

8 things you should know

Herpes is not a new disease. The Roman emperor Tiberius tried to stamp it out by banning kissing and Shakespeare wrote about it in *Romeo and Juliet*.

There are two types of herpes—herpes simplex 1 (HSV1) and herpes simplex 2 (HSV2) – but there are many different strains of the viruses. Both types of virus can infect either the mouth or the genital area and although herpes can be transmitted sexually it can also be transmitted in other ways. It is possible to get herpes more than once—because of the existence of different types of virus.

The first symptoms of a herpes infection can appear up to thirty years after the virus first arrived on the skin—an infected mother washing her child can give it herpes which does not erupt until half a lifetime later. The herpes HSV2 can live for seventy two hours on towels, clothing and lavatory seats.

The incidence of herpes is still increasing very rapidly. Ironically the increase is at least partly due to improving social conditions. A generation or two ago most people acquired immunity to herpes when they were exposed to the infection as children but these days we rarely share baths or towels with one another and so we grow up without ever being exposed to the herpes viruses. As a result we do not develop any immunity to them and are far more vulnerable when we reach adulthood.

Babies are the other group of people most at risk. Half the babies who die of herpes acquire the infection from their mothers and the other half from visitors or nurses. If a pregnant woman has active herpes the danger can be minimised by delivering her baby by Caesarian section.

The first symptoms of sexually transmitted herpes usually appear gradually. A few days, perhaps a week after sexual contact with someone carrying the infection, the sufferer will feel a little tired. He may have a fever and a headache and may also suffer from stiffness and backache. As these general symptoms develop so more specific symptoms will appear. There will be some local genital irritation and very probably a discharge. There may also be pain or burning when urine is passed. About four days after the onset of the irritation small blisters will probably appear on the penis or around the vagina and these may well be extremely sore. The glands in the groin will usually swell too.

Severe recurrences of herpes are relatively rare and around a third of sufferers have just one attack and no more. Another third of sufferers get occasional, infrequent and relatively minor outbreaks. Only a third of herpes sufferers get troublesome recurrences—and those are usually less painful than the initial attacks.

Things to remember about herpes:

1   Avoid having sex when a herpes lesion is visible.

2   Wash your hands carefully after visiting the toilet.

3   Don't sit on the seats in public lavatories.

4   Be gentle during sex if you have herpes—trauma can bring back symptoms.

5   Use plenty of lubrication during sex to keep friction to a minimum.

6   A condom will provide some protection—as will barrier creams.

7   Don't kiss or touch cold sores or genital sores.

8   Remember that stress and anxiety can make herpes lesions worse.

9   See your doctor about possible treatments.

HICCUPS

3 favourite remedies

There are probably as many cures for hiccups as there are causes–hundreds! Although they can be annoying and embarrassing, hiccups aren't usually dangerous. They are caused by a sudden spasm of the diaphragm, the sheet of muscle which separates the chest from the abdomen, and usually go away within an hour at the most.

Babies hiccup a lot–even in the womb–because the nerve which controls the diaphragm isn't properly under control–but in children and adults the commonest causes are:

1 Eating too quickly.
2 Exercising too soon after a meal.
3 Swallowing something unusually hot or cold.
4 Being very nervous or stressed.

Since hiccups usually go away by themselves many remedies have gained a false reputation for effectiveness. But there are a number of 'old wives' remedies which do seem to work–probably by having a shock effect on the diaphragm or its nerves.

My three favourite remedies for hiccups are:

1 Make the patient sneeze by tickling his nose.
2 Get him to drink a glass of cold water without a break.
3 Get him to hold his breath and count to ten.

If none of these cures works, doctors can prescribe drugs that usually do the trick.

HIGH BLOOD PRESSURE

9 ways to keep blood pressure down

Every week thousands of patients visit their doctor and discover they've got high blood pressure.

If high blood pressure isn't properly controlled then it can kill. It can, for example, produce strokes and heart attacks.

Look at these facts:

- At the age of 35 a man with a normal blood pressure can expect to live until the age of 76. But a man with a slightly raised blood pressure can expect to live only to the age of 60.

- At the age of 45 a woman with a normal blood pressure can expect to live until she is 82. But a woman with a slightly raised blood pressure can expect to live until she's 73.

Some high blood pressure sufferers will need to take pills for life to keep their blood pressure down.

If you are a high blood pressure sufferer you may be able to get your blood pressure back to normal–and keep it down–by following the advice below. First, however, it is important to tell your doctor what you are going to do. His help and support is essential because as your blood pressure comes down your pills may need changing. You will need to see your doctor at least once a month–and maybe more often.

1 Reduce your intake of salt. Avoid adding salt when you are cooking. Banish the salt cellar from the table. Cut down your consumption of crisps, salted peanuts, cheese, crackers, sausages, bacon, salted butter, canned foods and junk food.

2 Increase your intake of potassium by eating plenty of fresh fruit and vegetables.

3 Stop smoking–if you can't stop then cut down.

4 Drink less coffee and tea–or drink it weaker. Try decaffeinated coffee. If you drink ground coffee change to instant (which contains far less caffeine).

5 If you eat meat, reduce the amount of animal fat you eat. Cut down eggs, butter, milk and cream–and cut down fatty meat. Grill rather than fry, and cook with vegetable oils.

6 Lose any excess weight. Successful dieting will make a dramatic difference to your blood pressure.

7 Learn how to relax. Try not to let yourself get too excited too often. Organise your life to reduce your exposure to stress.

8 Take regular, gentle exercise: e.g. spend 30 minutes a day walking.

9   Control the amount of alcohol you drink. Limit yourself to 2 or 3 ordinary sized drinks a day at most.

HOME NURSING

10 tips to help patient and nurse

Here are some tips that will help make things easier for you (and the patient) if anyone in your family needs looking after at home.

1   Few patients need to stay in bed all day. Unless the doctor has given instructions to the contrary your patient should be able to get out of bed to bath and use the toilet. Most patients feel better if they are allowed to get up, watch TV or sit in a chair.

2   If you do have to look after a patient who is going to be bed–bound, try to get hold of a hospital–type bed. They're much higher that ordinary beds. Bending over an ordinary divan for more than a few days will soon give you a bad back.

3   Sick rooms soon get stuffy. Don't be afraid to have a window open. Germs like stale air.

4   Try to change sheets as often as you can. Crisp, clean bed sheets are wonderful. Powdering with talc helps to prevent the development of bed sores in long term patients.

5   If your patient needs to take pills keep a chart by the bed and tick off pills and medicine when they're given. That way you won't be left wondering whether or not you have given the right dose at the right time.

6   Patients often have poor appetites. Try to make food as attractive as possible. Don't put too much on the plate at once. Remember that weak patients are often better off with foods that don't need too much chewing or cutting.

7   If you need help or advice ask your doctor to arrange for a district nurse to call. She'll be able to offer expert, profes-sional advice and maybe lend you useful equipment.

8   To save too many journeys up and down the stairs fill a

vacuum flask with an iced drink and keep it by the bed.

9   Try to fix up some sort of communication system. Even a
    walking stick that can be banged on the floor is better than
    nothing.

10 Give your patient things to look forward to. Point out good
    programmes on the TV or radio. Keep a few magazines,
    books, puzzles etc. on one side for really dull moments. And
    although visitors can be a help remember that too many
    visitors can be tiring!

HORMONE REPLACEMENT THERAPY (HRT)

☞ *See* Menopause.

HYPERACTIVITY

How to find out if your child is hyperactive

Children who suffer from hyperactivity find it difficult to keep
quiet and still for more than a few moments at a time. They are
over–excitable, disruptive and difficult to control. They are
often reckless as well as restless and can wreck a room in five
minutes. As many as one in ten children may suffer from hyperactivity and it is a condition that is well known to school
teachers and playgroups leaders as well as thousands of parents.
It is sometimes difficult to differentiate between children who
are merely mischievous and children who are truly hyperactive.

A hyperactive child will be moving virtually all the time. He
won't be able to sit still and watch TV, play games or read. His
behaviour will be annoying and disturbing for everyone. And
he really won't be able to help himself.

No one really knows exactly what makes some children
hyperactive. But food additives are widely recognised as being
responsible for many cases of hyperactivity and thousands of
children who suffer from hyperactivity have been helped by
cutting down on the consumption of additives.

There is a fairly simple test you can do to find out if your child's behaviour could be a result of something in his food. You should only try this test after you have consulted your doctor and obtained his permission.

For one whole week cut out all sweet and sugary foods from his diet. At the same time give him plenty of fresh and dried fruit, fresh vegetables, nuts, diluted unsweetened fresh fruit juice, wholemeal bread and savoury spreads. Then, after the week is up, let him go back to his normal diet and see if you notice any changes. Make sure that your doctor knows and approves of what you are doing.

HYSTERECTOMY

4 facts women should know

Hysterectomy—the surgical removal of the womb—is by far the commonest major operation performed on women. Every year tens of thousands of women have the operation—it is estimated that roughly one in three women will eventually have a hysterectomy.

Many women who have the operation understand very little about it. Some worry that they will stop being 'proper' women. They assume that they will grow old suddenly, that their sex lives will stop and that they will suffer a wide range of symptoms.

Here are some facts about hysterectomy.

1   Women having a hysterectomy usually need to stay in hospital for between 10 and 14 days. They usually need to stay off work for 4–6 weeks.

2   Up to half of all hysterectomies are done to stop bleeding caused by benign (harmless) fibroids or by a hormonal imbalance. Only a relatively small number are done because of cancer. The operation may also be performed to treat a severe and uncontrollable infection, in an attempt to treat period pains which cannot be controlled in any other way or to treat a prolapse.

3   Traditionally there are two ways to remove a uterus. A cut

can be made vertically or horizontally in the abdomen (if the cut is horizontal it can usually be hidden by bikini bottoms). The uterus can then be removed through the opening. Alternatively, the womb can be removed through the vagina. This technique sounds—and is—more difficult so it's done less often. But it leaves no scar.

4   After the op women need to avoid sex for 4–6 weeks to give their tissues time to heal. After that there should be no problem. One major study showed that 94% of women reported that their sex lives were *better* after a hysterectomy. They said that sex was less painful and more enjoyable and they liked not having to worry about pregnancy. The one problem reported after a hysterectomy is that the vagina may become a little drier than before. A little artificial lubrication will sort this out.

Note: Far too many surgeons remove wombs in order to make money (it is a widely performed 'private' operation that is well known as a 'money–spinner' in medical circles). I strongly suggest that any woman who is told that she needs a hysterectomy ask her doctor why she needs to have it done and if there are any alternatives.

IMPOTENCE

10 causes and 8 tips for sufferers

Most—probably all—men are impotent at one time or another and impotence always seems to be the end of the world to a previously virile male. It usually (and perhaps inevitably) strikes at the most inopportune and most embarrassing moment. It certainly strikes at a moment when a man is most vulnerable.

The symptoms are simple: he cannot acquire an erection easily and/or if he does get one then it is either too feeble or too short lived to enable him to penetrate his partner.

Here are some of the most likely causes of impotence.

1   ANXIETY Anxiety about failure is a common cause of impotence. The risk of failure is proportional to the build

up. If a man really wants to impress his partner then the chances of his being impotent are high. Men who worry about how well they are doing are also prone to impotence.

2 TIREDNESS Tiredness, often through overwork, is a common cause of impotence.

3 FEAR A man will have difficulty in acquiring an erection if he is frightened of catching a disease, of being caught, of making his partner pregnant, of hurting her or causing himself pain.

4 OBESITY Men who are fat are more likely to suffer from impotence.

5 INADEQUACY Some men feel very inadequate about their bodies, not simply about the size or shape of their penises. This can lead to impotence.

6 ALCOHOL Alcohol and tobacco can cause impotence.

7 DISEASE Diabetes can cause impotence.

8 GUILT A married man who tries to make love to a woman other than his wife will be prone to impotence.

9 MEMORIES A man who tries to make love in a room or bed he associates with someone else may suffer from impotence.

10 DRUGS Some prescribed drugs can sometimes cause impotence.

Age does not really figure on the list of possible causes. Age can affect the amount of time a man must wait for his second erection but it is not itself a cause of impotence.

Next, some tips for the man suffering from impotence.

1 If you do occasionally get an erection (asleep or awake, alone or with a partner) then there is nothing wrong with your equipment. The problem is in your mind and can be conquered. The vast majority of cases of impotence fit into this category.

2 The more you worry about the problem the worse it will get.

3 If you are totally unable to have an erection at any time then your problem may need treatment with hormones. Talk to your doctor.

4   You must slowly and gradually rebuild your confidence. You should try to deal with any anxieties or problems in other parts of your life and you should spend a little time learning how to relax.

5   You will find it easier to conquer your impotence if you have a regular partner rather than a number of occasional partners or a succession of one night stands. With new partners you will have to explain your problem repeatedly and will undoubtedly find it more stressful.

6   Spend time on foreplay. Learn how to please your partner in ways other than full intercourse. If you know that you can bring your partner to orgasm before you have entered her then the pressure on you will be reduced enormously. Try to relax with your partner as often as you can—and to cuddle and kiss frequently.

7   Some experts recommend that men who are suffering from impotence should make a decision to try not to have sex for six weeks. During that time, they say, you should concentrate on touching your partner. You should become adept at foreplay. Even if you have an erection you should not have sex. You should learn to relax and enjoy your partner. Bring her to orgasm with your hands and encourage her to do the same for you. If, after six weeks, you are regularly getting erections then you can make love. If not, you should extend your period of deliberate abstinence for another four weeks. Taking the pressure off in this way can work wonders.

8   Finally, if your erection is a weak one you will find that penetration is far easier to achieve if you lie side by side or if your partner sits on top of you. The missionary position is not good for men who suffer from partial impotence.

INDIGESTION

10 tips for sufferers

The word indigestion simply means that there has been a failure of digestion and so it can theoretically refer to a small intestine problem as well as a stomach problem. The word 'dyspepsia' is often used as an alternative to 'indigestion'. In practice, the word 'indigestion' is used to describe the sort of symptoms which occur when a meal is eaten too quickly or after an unusually spicy or fatty meal. Sufferers usually complain of some pain in the centre of the chest. They may also feel slightly bloated. It's common for indigestion sufferers to complain of excessive wind and nausea. Occasionally they will actually vomit. Very few people who have indigestion will be interested in food for the pain tends to be accompanied by a full feeling and a loss of appetite.

Indigestion can be caused by smoking too much, by drinking too much alcohol or by taking too much tea or coffee. Other drugs, such as aspirin, can also cause indigestion.

However, although these specific causes are significant, many of the individuals who suffer from indigestion do so directly as a result of stress.

Heartburn

Under normal circumstances the acid mixture that helps to digest food within the stomach is kept away from the oesophagus by a sphincter which allows food to travel down into the stomach but doesn't allow food and acid to travel upwards into the gullet. If the sphincter which usually divides the oesophagus from the stomach in this way doesn't do its job properly, acid can sometimes splash upwards and irritate the oesophageal mucosa (stomach lining). The word 'heartburn' is very descriptive. Even when the sphincter is in good working condition, acid can irritate the oesophagus when you lie down or bend over. Naturally enough, therefore, individuals who have a weak sphincter at that point will find that they suffer far more when they are lying flat or bending over than they do when they are standing up straight.

Despite the fact that heartburn can have a solid physical cause there are many individuals who suffer from this symptom purely as a result of stress.

Gastritis

Gastritis is an inflammation of the stomach that can be produced by alcohol, by the consumption of a foodstuff to which you are allergic, by a virus infection or by any one of a number of other mechanisms which are not yet properly understood. There are some specific changes in the stomach lining when gastritis is present, but in practice it is virtually impossible to differentiate clinically between dyspepsia, gastritis and peptic ulceration without undergoing specific investigations such as a barium meal examination or an endoscopy.

Peptic ulcer

The terms peptic ulcer, gastric ulcer and duodenal ulcer are often used as though they are completely interchangeable. In fact, however, there are differences. A peptic ulcer is simply any ulcer in the upper part of the intestinal tract. The word 'peptic' is used as a synonym for digestion. A gastric ulcer is one that is found in the stomach, while a duodenal ulcer is one that is found in the duodenum. The phrase 'peptic ulceration' can be used to describe either a stomach ulcer or a duodenal ulcer.

Ulcers of all kinds result from an imbalance between the power of the secretions produced by the stomach and the resistance of the lining of the part of the intestine concerned.

Gastric ulcer

We still really don't know precisely what causes a gastric ulcer or why the acid suddenly starts to eat away at the stomach lining to produce an ulcer cavity. What we do know is that although individuals who have gastric ulcers don't seem to be producing more acid than other people they do have a weaker stomach lining.

There is also evidence that the stomach lining can be damaged by a number of different factors—tobacco, alcohol and fats, for example. This explains why individuals who have gastric ulcers will usually get better quicker if they cut out cigarettes and alcohol and if they steer away from fatty foods as much as possible. Gastric ulcer pain is usually localised to the epigastrium, a central point about half way between the chin and the navel, and eating usually makes it worse. Unlike duodenal ulcer pain, gastric ulcer pain doesn't usually go away once it has started.

Duodenal ulcer

Scientists still have not yet decided precisely how duodenal ulcers develop, but it is widely believed that they result from some imbalance between the power of the stomach's acid secretions to attack and the ability of the duodenal lining to resist the attack. It is a fine balance and one that can fairly easily be tipped one way or the other. The most important symptom of a duodenal ulcer is usually pain, and indeed this is often the only symptom that occurs. The pain is usually localised in the epigastrium (see above), and unlike with gastric ulcers, eating usually helps relieve the pain, albeit temporarily. People who have duodenal ulcers will often wake up at night and sneak downstairs to get a glass of milk and a biscuit. The other characteristic of the pain with duodenal ulceration is that it tends to disappear for weeks or even months at a time for no very apparent reason. Suddenly, just when you thought it had gone away for ever, back it comes with a bang!

How to look after your stomach

Most of us have a weak point. Some people get headaches when they are under pressure. Others get asthma, heart pains, diarrhoea or skin rashes. The human body, like most complex pieces of machinery, doesn't go all wrong at once. There is usually one part that is weaker than the rest. If you are a regular sufferer from indigestion, ulcer pains or other stomach symptoms, the chances are that your stomach is your weak point. Make sure you see your doctor and tell him all your symptoms.

You can do a lot to look after your stomach and keep it healthy. To begin with it is a good idea to learn to listen to your stomach and to get into the habit of eating when you are hungry rather than just because the clock tells you that it is time to eat. You may not know it but you have an appetite control centre which is designed to control your eating habits quite accurately.

Research studies showed that young children automatically chose foods that enabled them to avoid digestive upsets and constipation. Other studies, done on soldiers during the Second World War, showed that when allowed access to unlimited supplies of food, troops ate what their bodies needed according to the outside temperature. They automatically chose an ideal mixture of protein, fat and carbohydrate.

Unfortunately, most of us have lost the art of listening to our own bodies and we tend to eat three meals a day whether we are hungry or not, stuffing our bodies with food not because we need it but because the clock says it is time to eat. In practice the stomach does not adapt well to huge meals at lengthy intervals and it can cope far more effectively with smaller meals taken at shorter intervals.

We've also lost the art of knowing when we've had enough to eat. Most of us make the mistake of always finishing the food on our plates because we've been trained that wasting food is wrong. Your stomach will be much healthier (and far less likely to succumb to stress) if you re-establish control of your appetite control centre by eating when you feel hungry, stopping when you feel full—and nibbling smaller meals more frequently rather than stuffing yourself with large meals occasionally.

Rules for healthier eating

1   Eat slowly. People often stuff food into their mouths at an unbelievable rate when they are under stress. A medical friend of mine used to be spooning up the last smear of custard while the rest of us were still finishing our soup. He always had indigestion afterwards and had to sit for half an hour to allow the pain to disappear.

2   Don't try eating while you're reading or watching television. A little mild and gentle conversation probably won't do much harm but you should concentrate as much as you can when you're eating. Only by concentrating on what you are doing will you become able to tell when your stomach is talking to you. If you listen your stomach will tell you when you're eating something that is going to upset you, or eating too much.

3   Try and put small forkfuls into your mouth. Stuff huge

amounts of food onto your fork and you'll end up failing to chew your food properly. Chewing is an essential part of the digestive process and the saliva in your mouth contains enzymes which help prepare your food for the secretions produced by the stomach.

4 Try to taste each mouthful of food that you eat. That way you're far less likely to eat unnecessarily or too quickly.

5 If you are a fast eater put down your knife and fork between mouthfuls. That will slow you down effectively.

6 Don't let other people push you into eating when you aren't hungry or when you don't want a second helping. And do be prepared to leave food on the side of your plate if you've had enough to eat.

7 Remember that regular meals are better for you than irregular meals. By eating regularly you'll be helping to mop up some of the acid in your stomach. If you eat irregularly the acid in your stomach will have nothing to get its teeth into.

8 When you've finished a meal have a short rest. Give your stomach time to do its job before you start chasing around again.

9 Try to find out what sort of foods upset your stomach most —and avoid them. Different people are badly affected by different foods, so it is impossible to offer a comprehensive list of foods to avoid, but if you do have a 'weak' stomach it is likely that any of the foods on the list below will exacerbate your symptoms:

- All fried foods
- Strong tea or coffee
- Fizzy drinks
- Alcohol
- Fatty foods
- Spicy foods
- Pickles, curry, peppers, mustard
- Broad beans, brussels sprouts, radishes and cucumber

- Unripe fruit
- Very hot or very cold foods or drinks
- Coarse bread, biscuits or cereals
- Nuts or dried fruit
- Any tough food that can't be chewed easily

You do not have to avoid all these foods if you have stomach symptoms. But do be aware that these foods can cause problems. The important thing is to find out which foods upset you and avoid them. Do remember that when and how you eat probably affects your stomach more than what you eat.

10   Give up smoking. We don't know very much about the ways in which peptic ulcers develop but we do know that tobacco smoke irritates the lining of the stomach and makes it more vulnerable to attack by acid. All stomach sufferers will, therefore, find that they suffer far less if they can give up smoking.

☞ *See also* Wind.

INSOMNIA

☞ *See* Sleeplessness.

IRRITABLE BOWEL SYNDROME

Symptoms and 4 solutions

Most irritable bowel syndrome sufferers complain of several symptoms.

The primary symptoms are those which involve the bowel itself and what goes on inside it. Pain is probably the most obvious of these symptoms – though it is also one of the most variable. It is often a colicky, spasmodic sort of pain which comes and goes in waves; it can affect just about any part of the abdomen and it frequently fades a little when the sufferer goes to the toilet. Bowel irregularities are common too. Most sufferers complain of diarrhoea—which can sometimes be quite sudden and explosive—though, oddly enough, constipation is also a common symptom. Sometimes the two problems alternate. Most sufferers also complain of wind.

In a survey of irritable bowel syndrome sufferers which was published in the *British Medical Journal* recently it was found that every single patient with this problem complained of these three symptoms: (1) abdominal pain, (2) abdominal distension caused by wind, and (3) an abnormal bowel habit.

Next, there are the secondary symptoms which affect a lot of sufferers but which don't affect all patients. One or two of the secondary symptoms are caused by the wind that is so widely associated with the irritable bowel syndrome and these will probably come and go as the wind comes and goes. Symptoms in this category include a feeling of being full all the time and not being able to eat very much, a constant feeling of nausea, heartburn and indigestion. Back pains of one sort or another are also fairly commonplace and these too are frequently a result of wind accumulating in the intestines. It's even quite common for irritable bowel syndrome sufferers to complain of having to pass urine more often than usual because of pressure produced by wind in the intestines.

Last, but certainly not least, there are the mental symptoms which aren't in any direct way related to the intestines or what is going on inside them. Anxiety, depression and irritability are all common but the one mental symptom that really seems to affect irritable bowel syndrome patients more than any other is tiredness.

Even though you may be quite convinced that you are suffering from the irritable bowel syndrome you shouldn't make the diagnosis by yourself without visiting your doctor. Although it is probably the commonest of all bowel problems today there are other problems which can cause bowel symptoms and only by visiting your doctor can you be absolutely sure that you have got the diagnosis right.

There are two main causes of the irritable bowel syndrome. The first is stress. All muscles can be tightened up by stress.

Tension headaches are a good example of what happens when the muscles around the head are tightened by worry and anxiety. The muscles in the bowel walls are no exception—they are as vulnerable and as susceptible to stress as any other muscles—and in some individuals it is these muscles which suffer first when stress starts to get out of control. Lots of people who don't suffer from the irritable bowel syndrome do get diarrhoea or cramping pains in their tummies when they are under too much pressure or when they are anxious.

The second explanation for the current epidemic of irritable bowel syndrome lies in the type of food we tend to eat these days. Most of us tend to eat a bland over–refined diet that contains very little natural roughage. And the result is that our bowels can't cope very well with this change—they haven't had time to adapt and so they struggle. We tend to live on prepackaged, convenience foods that may be rich in vitamins and minerals but which are dangerously short on fibre.

There is no single wonder cure for the irritable bowel syndrome but there are a good many ways in which you can control your symptoms.

1   There are some pills which your doctor may want to prescribe which could help you enormously. If you suffer a lot from colicky spasms of pain then an anti–spasmodic drug may be a real boon. There are several useful drugs available. If the two symptoms which worry you most are pain and wind, peppermint oil capsules may be helpful. If diarrhoea is your most troublesome symptom, your doctor can choose from several suitable drugs. If constipation is more of a worry—and some patients who suffer from the irritable bowel syndrome do suffer from both diarrhoea and constipation at different times—your doctor may decide to prescribe something called a 'bulking agent' to help give your stools more substance.

2   Take a good, hard look at the amount of stress in your life. Try, for example, to make a list of all the things which worry you, which make you feel uptight, which keep you awake at night, which give you butterflies in your stomach

or which you know upset you. Try to decide what things are really important to you. Decide how you are going to allocate your time. And make sure that every week you take some time off. If you want to relax properly you're going to have to work at it—and that will take a little effort and a little time. Learning to relax is like learning to drive a car or learning to play golf or learning to dance: you'll only get good at it if you put some effort into it.

3   Take a long, cool, careful and critical look at your diet. You will almost certainly benefit if you gradually increase the amount of fibre that you eat. To do this start eating whole-meal bread or high bran cereals. Eat wholewheat pasta, brown rice, oats—in porridge for example—and more fresh vegetables and fruit, though if you suffer a lot from wind you will probably be wise to avoid any vegetables—such as sprouts—which seem to cause you a lot of wind. Nibble fruit and nuts instead of chocolate and sweets and eat plenty of pulses. Try to cut down your fat intake too. If you eat meat, cut off the visible fat and avoid red meats as often as you can. If you drink milk, drink skimmed milk rather than the full fat variety. Buy low fat salad dressings. You may find that your condition is a lot easier if you avoid dairy products completely. Make low fat pastry; don't add fat when cooking; and grill, bake, steam, poach, casserole and boil rather than roast or fry. When you make chips cut them thickly so that they soak up less fat and make sure that the fat is sizzling hot. Replace butter on vegetables with herbs and instead of butter on bread use a low fat spread.

4   Try to do more exercise. Don't make the mistake of adding stress to your life by trying to run faster than anyone else or by trying to win the local tennis club trophy. But do try to take more exercise that is fun. Walk, swim, dance, cycle or work out in the gym—all those things will help you because gentle, regular exercise seems to have a soothing effect on the bowel.

ITCHING

When someone has an itch, it's because the nerve endings in his skin have been stimulated—by something he has eaten, by an insect, by clothes or by stress. The nerves are stimulated by irritating chemicals produced by the body. When the sufferer scratches the area he damages the nerve endings and substitutes the sensation of pain for the itch. Amazingly most of us find this mild pain preferable to the itch!

But the snag is that the scratching stimulates the body to produce another batch of irritating chemicals—which can bring the itching back a few minutes later. The best answer is to soothe the skin with a moisturising cream—or with calamine lotion.

☞ *See also* Eczema.

JAUNDICE

Jaundice is a symptom rather than a disease. The word simply denotes that the skin is yellow, usually as a result of the deposition of bile pigments in the tissues. These pigments come from the breakdown of old red blood cells.

The skin and the eyes go yellow as a result of the accumulation of the pigment bilirubin in the blood. The urine goes dark.

Normally the bile pigments are turned into bile, carried via the bile ducts into the intestines and then discarded.

Jaundice can develop:

- If a blood disease means that red blood cells are broken down faster than the liver can cope with them.
- If an infection (such as hepatitis) or any other disease which affects the organ means that the liver is unable to function properly.
- If an obstruction—such as a trapped gallstone—prevents bile from flowing from the liver into the intestines.

JET LAG

10 practical tips

The longer your flight the more likely you are to suffer problems. Flights going eastwards usually seem to cause more problems that flights travelling westward.

1   Unless you cannot survive without a cigarette avoid the smoking section on planes. Smoke will dry out your sinuses, affect your eyes and produce a variety of other symptoms. The air inside a plane is already unusually dry—smoke makes it worse.

2   Avoid heavy meals before and during travel. Light snacks are much better for you.

3   Avoid drinks such as tea and coffee which contain caffeine. Flying tends to cause dehydration and caffeine makes this worse.

4   If you are flying at night take ear plugs and a mask with you and try to sleep during the flight.

5   Drink lots of water or fruit juice during the flight—that's what pilots do to help them keep fresh and alert. Avoid alcohol—it's likely to make you feel worse.

6   Use plenty of moisturising cream on your skin before flying. The dry air inside a plane can make the skin dry and itchy.

7   Suck peppermints during your flight. The pressure inside aircraft cabins is low and this means that any gas inside your intestines will expand. This can be very painful. Peppermint helps to reduce the pain and discomfort.

8   If you suffer from sinus troubles or have a cold, swallow frequently to even out the pressure in your sinuses.

9   Try to get up and walk about once an hour on long flights. If you can't do that then at least make sure that you move your feet and legs at regular intervals to help keep blood moving around your body. Blood clots are among the commonest cause of death among travellers—and sitting still for long periods makes them more likely.

10 Make no plans at all for the first 24 hours after your plane touches down. Just take things easy. Keep strenuous, exciting or demanding activities for later in your trip.

LEFT HANDEDNESS

Many investigators have tried to find out just what causes left–handedness but there is still no conclusive evidence. There may be links to breech births or to babies born to mothers over the age of 38. The condition can be inherited and although there does seem to be a genetic link it is not possible to forecast whether or not a child will be left–handed. More boys than girls are left–handed.

The condition is not linked to any other physical or mental problems. It was often thought that left–handedness was linked to stuttering, but this is now thought to be almost certainly due to the anxiety at being 'different' felt by the children concerned. If your child chooses to use his left hand when playing or picking up objects then the chances are that he is left–handed. Do not try to make him change hands—this will produce anxiety and may slow down his development.

LOW BLOOD PRESSURE

5 symptoms and 3 cures

Many doctors fail to take low blood pressure seriously because in its mild, common form it never leads to death. But it may be the failure of the drug companies to find a profitable cure that has really made low blood pressure an unfashionable diagnosis. Some doctors and drug companies feel comfortable with illnesses that can't be cured by pills.

Low blood pressure can, however, cause devastating and disruptive symptoms that can ruin a sufferer's life.

The vast majority of sufferers are women—thin and rather 'delicately' built.

The symptoms are:

1   General weakness and lack of stamina.

2   Cold hands and feet.

3   Difficulty in getting up and 'getting going' in the morning.

4   Persistent, mild depression.

5   Dizziness, particularly when getting up or moving around.

In addition many sufferers will have been told by their doctors that they have low blood pressure.

Every time the heart contracts it puts the 10 pints of blood lying in the arteries and veins under pressure. That pressure pushes fresh oxygen-carrying blood to the brain, stomach, arms and legs. If the pressure is too high there's a risk that a blood vessel will burst, producing a stroke. But if the pressure is too low the result will be a feeling of tiredness and dizziness because the brain and muscles won't be getting the supplies they need.

Patients with low blood pressure can treat themselves in three ways.

1   Exercise. Firming up the muscles and making your tissues demand oxygen seems to help. Ideally you should join a gym where you can try mild weight lifting and gentle aerobic exercises such as jogging and cycling. Start gently to begin with or you may feel dizzy and faint. But after a week or two you should notice that you have more energy and 'get up and go'. Do not start an exercise programme without talking first to your doctor.

2   Cool showers. Your circulating blood responds quickly and dramatically to the temperature of your skin. So one way to stimulate your circulation is to take a cool shower. You should find that this makes you feel livelier!

3   Put more stress into your life. Stress and pressure can push up the blood pressure of an ordinary individual to dangerous levels. But if your blood pressure is normally low you may find that you benefit—and feel fresher—if you deliberately add a little more stress to your life. If your job is relatively quiet and undemanding try taking up a hobby or sport that challenges you. Instead of slumping down in front of the TV go to an evening class or for a swim. But do talk to your doctor first and clear your plans with him.

MEASLES

Measles is a very common virus infection which occurs in minor, local epidemics. The symptoms are usually those of a cold—slight temperature, a sniffle and a cough—and possibly some inflammation of the eyes. On the third day the rash begins, usually starting on the neck at the back of the head. Small red spots clump together to form red blotches which appear all over the body. The measles rash is not itchy and by the time the whole body is covered the patient may seem quite well.

Measles is very infectious and is spread by touch or breath. After contact with an infected person the patient will take 1—2 weeks to develop symptoms. He can pass the infection on before his own rash develops and will remain infectious until a week after the rash disappears.

Treatment usually involves sponging with tepid water to relieve any fever. Sore eyes should be protected from bright lights.

Most people with measles do not need medical attention. If however, the patient suffers ear pains, vomits or has a headache then you should get in touch with your doctor. Occasional complications do develop with measles and so any unusual symptoms should be seen by a doctor.

M.E. (MYALGIC ENCEPHALOMYELITIS)

☞ *See* Tiredness.

MEDICINE CABINET

What to put in it

Every home should have a medicine cabinet which is properly stocked. Ideally the medicine cabinet should have a lock on it so that the medicines inside can be kept out of the reach of small children. However, it is also sensible to put the medicine cabinet in a position where children cannot get hold of it—just in case it is left open.

Although medicine cabinets are traditionally kept in the bathroom this really isn't the best place for drugs: the variations in temperature which occur may accelerate the rate at which drugs deteriorate. Any room—such as a bedroom—which has a more or less stable temperature is much more suitable.

Take everything out of your medicine cabinet and examine each packet and bottle carefully. Throw away anything which is improperly labelled. Throw out any medicine which is over six months old. Throw away anything which you aren't entirely sure how—and when—to use properly.

Your medicine cabinet should contain:

- A pain reliever such as soluble aspirin or paracetamol
- A hot water bottle—an excellent treatment for aching muscles and joints
- A small bottle of liquid antiseptic for cleaning cuts and grazes
- A bottle of calamine lotion to help with itchy rashes
- A bottle of menthol crystals to help relieve catarrh and sinus troubles
- A bottle of indigestion mixture (ask your local pharmacist to recommend something suitable)
- A thermometer (make sure you know how to use it)
- A packet of fabric sticking plasters
- A measuring spoon for medicines
- An eye bath
- Whatever bandages you can use without tying yourself up in knots
- Moisturising cream for dry skin

MEMORY

10 ways to improve your memory

The parts of your brain which are responsible for remembering things like dates, recipes, names and addresses, telephone numbers and directions lose up to 100,000 nerve cells a day.

Teenagers are better able to absorb and remember pages of

information than adults. If you're older than 25 then your medium term memory is slowly getting worse and worse.

However, just as medium term memory deteriorates with age so mental ability to use information increases.

Your memory may be failing as you age but you are becoming wiser. People under 25 may be better able to remember lists of equations and irregular verbs. But the best thinking in any society is done by the over 25s.

Still, there is no doubt that it is inconvenient to have a deteriorating memory. So here are a few ways in which you can improve your memory and disguise the fact that you are getting older.

1 As your brain gets older so your ability to remember things that you have looked at briefly will get worse. When you were young you could probably look at a list of words and remember quite a lot of them. You can't do that as easily when you're older. You need to concentrate more. To remember where you parked the car you will need to make a conscious effort. Look at your car and its surroundings to imprint the view on your memory. Pretend that you are taking a photograph of it—blink your eyelids as though your eyes were cameras—and you'll remember it better.

2 Normally we remember around 20% of what we read. But if you really concentrate you can remember up to 70%. After reading something that you want to remember spend 60 seconds thinking about it. Make a mental comment to yourself about what you have read. Rephrase it in your mind. You will find that if you do this your memory will improve considerably.

3 As we get older we all do things without really thinking about them. We put ourselves onto 'automatic pilot' and fall into a routine. Concentrate really hard and spot the things you do without thinking. Then ask yourself whether or not you could do things better if you thought about them more.

4 Try to understand things that you have to remember. You will find things easier to remember if you understand them.

And try to remember key facts and key words which will help bring into your mind whole sequences of thoughts and facts.

5   Clear your brain of trivial information. Use notebooks and diaries to record trivial material. Albert Einstein once said: 'Why should I waste brain space remembering my own telephone number? I can look it up if I want to know what it is.'

6   When you are talking about something you know that you will want to remember, try to concentrate hard on everything around you. Concentrate on the people you are with and the place you are in. Try to be aware of smells, sights and sounds. The more information you record the easier you will find it to remember the event.

7   When you are trying to remember something do your best to recreate the conditions under which you learnt it. Football teams do best when playing at home (even if there isn't a crowd of home supporters) because they find it easier to remember what they've learned while training. Students do better in examinations if they take their tests in the room where they did their learning. So, if you are trying to remember the name of someone you met at a party, try to remember where you were, what you were doing, what you were wearing, what other people were wearing and what you said to the people you met. Things that you learn are bound together in your mind in time and place. If you can recreate the conditions in which you learned something then your ability to recall the facts will increase dramatically.

8   If you are struggling to remember something work your way through the alphabet. The first letter of a name or place can often 'trigger' a lost memory.

9   If you want to remember something that you have seen or read try closing your eyes immediately afterwards. This keeps the 'image' on your retina for a little longer—and will make the image easier to recall in the future.

10   To make it easier to remember names try to make up pictures in your mind. For example, to remember the name 'Coleman' think of a man carrying a bag of coal. If you are

trying to remember a name like 'Vernon' which doesn't lend itself to a picture, visualise an imaginary blackboard in your mind and then write the name onto your blackboard. When you want to recall the name simply recreate your blackboard.

MENINGITIS

Symptoms to watch out for

Meningitis, an infection and inflammation of the membranes (or meninges—hence the name of the disease) which cover the brain and the spinal cord, is a killer disease.

Several different types of bug can cause the disease.

- Viral meningitis is often over in a week or two and isn't usually particularly dangerous.
- Bacterial meningitis can be much more deadly. Even with modern treatment—usually needing large doses of antibiotic drugs given intravenously—as many as one in five sufferers with some types of infection may die.

Meningitis can be a complication of an ear or throat infection but any infection which gets into the blood stream can eventually reach the brain. Most commonly the bugs that can cause meningitis can be spread by mouth or hand—just like the bugs which can cause coughs and colds. It is a very infectious disease. Some individuals can carry the disease for months—getting no symptoms themselves but passing it on to others.

Initially the symptoms can appear mild and are often mistaken for flu—but they can get worse frighteningly quickly. Indeed, it is the speed with which meningitis develops that makes it so dangerous. Many doctors regard it as one of the most dramatic emergencies in medicine. One minute a patient may be feeling a little unwell—with a fever and a headache. Within hours he will begin to get a stiff neck and a dislike of bright lights. When the meninges are infected they irritate the brain tissue—causing delirium, confusion and a dramatically enhanced sensitivity to light and noise. Within less than half a day of the first symptoms appearing he may be unconscious and close to death.

Even when meningitis doesn't kill it can cause serious after effects. Brain damage and deafness are just two of the problems that can develop.

Antibiotics can help to fight the infection but official information about the disease has been so restrained that parents and family doctors still miss the diagnosis—with devastating results.

In babies the symptoms of meningitis include:

1   Irritability or fretfulness

2   Loss of appetite or refusing feeds

3   Pale or blotchy skin

4   A rash—red or purple spots or bruises

5   High pitched or moaning cry

6   Vomiting

7   Fever

Few victims have all these symptoms. Most will get at least three.

In older children and adults, the main symptoms include:

1   Fever

2   Stiff neck

3   Severe headache

4   Nausea and vomiting

5   Eye discomfort in bright light

6   Pains in back and joints

7   Tiny red or purple rash or bruises

8   Drowsiness or confusion leading to unconsciousness

Again, few victims will have all these symptoms. But most will get at least three.

If you think that someone in your family could have meningitis, don't hesitate. Call your doctor immediately and insist that he takes the problem seriously. If you doctor can't or won't come straight away, take the patient to the nearest hospital that has a casualty department.

If the right antibiotic can be found quickly and the bug

causing the infection killed, the symptoms will disappear fast. But if the bug is tough several different antibiotics may be needed at once and finding the right combination can take time. Even when the bug is beaten the after effects may be dramatic. Roughly one in seven sufferers will get problems for many months, or even years. Depression, fits, hearing loss, giddiness, ringing in the ears, lack of coordination and general tiredness can all occur.

MENOPAUSE

Most women reach the menopause between the ages of 40 and 55. The production of sex hormones slows down, the ovaries stop producing eggs and monthly periods cease.

The problems associated with the menopause are largely to do with the fall in oestrogen levels. The symptoms can include: hot flushes and sweats, anxiety, irritability, depression, tiredness, sleeplessness, lowering of interest in sex, aches and pains, hair and skin changes, forgetfulness, loss of confidence, strange taste or burning in the mouth, incontinence, dry and sore vagina, an increased incidence of broken bones.

Specific treatments may be available for individual symptoms (such as giving calcium to strengthen bones) but the most successful treatment is hormone replacement therapy (HRT).

Ten things women should know about the menopause and hormone replacement therapy

1   It is not true that all women suffer unpleasant symptoms during the menopause! Many don't suffer any unpleasant symptoms at all. When they do, it is because their bodies are no longer producing so much oestrogen. The fall in oestrogen levels produces a variety of symptoms. The commonest are:

- hot flushes and sweats
- anxiety, depression, irritability and tiredness
- inability to sleep at night
- fall in sexual interest—and pain during intercourse

- aches and pains—headaches and joint pains in particular
- hair thinning and skin wrinkling
- dry and sore vagina
- urinary symptoms such as incontinence
- increased incidence of broken bones

The aim of HRT is artificially to replace the natural hormones which start to decline during the menopause. It doesn't prevent all the symptoms associated with the menopause—but it does help to combat some of the most important.

2 HRT is usually prescribed for a fairly long period of time if it is going to have a useful effect. It is common for women to take it for between 18 months and 2 years and not unusual for women to keep on HRT for 5 years. Women who are taking HRT to prevent the development of osteoporosis may need to take the tablets more or less indefinitely.

3 The vital hormone in HRT is oestrogen though many pills contain both oestrogen and progestogen because this reduces the risk of cancer of the uterus developing.

4 HRT is only available on a doctor's prescription. So if your doctor won't prescribe it for you the only way you can get it is either to persuade your doctor to refer you to a hospital specialist (in the hope that he will prescribe it for you) or to change to another family doctor! There are some patients for whom HRT is unsuitable. So, for example, it might be dangerous for you to take HRT if:

- you have a history of blood clots or you have had a heart attack or stroke
- you have high blood pressure
- you smoke heavily
- you have a history of liver disease
- you have had cancer
- there is a family history of cancer
- you have suffered from benign (harmless) breast or

womb lumps

• you suffer from undiagnosed vaginal bleeding

In all these instances taking HRT could be hazardous to your health.

5   There are quite a number of drug companies making HRT pills. Inevitably, therefore, there are a variety of different brand names. In addition doctors sometimes prescribe creams and pessaries containing oestrogen to help deal with some of the specific symptoms associated with the menopause.

6   One of the most useful qualities of HRT is that it can help control the thinning and weakening of the bones that often follows the menopause—and which is often responsible for fractures after fairly ordinary falls. Women who suffer from osteoporosis (the medical term for 'thin' and 'weak' bones) may need to take HRT for relatively long periods—e.g. for some years.

7   HRT is good at helping to stop hot flushes and reverse vaginal changes. It is also excellent at helping to prevent bone thinning. But it doesn't help to relieve emotional or psychological symptoms, nor does it do much to stop the effect of ageing on the skin. It does stop sweating quite effectively and it can help restore a woman's interest in sex—but it doesn't seem to do very much for symptoms such as tiredness, headaches and backache.

8   Most of the serious side effects associated with HRT can usually be avoided if doctors select the patients they give HRT to fairly carefully. Side effects can include nausea, breast tenderness, leg cramps and fluid retention. More serious problems include the possible risk of blood clotting and cancer (which is why some patients are not considered suitable for HRT).

9   Occasional bleeding does sometimes occur among women taking HRT. But any woman whose periods have stopped should always see her doctor for a check up if she notices any bleeding—whether or not she's taking HRT.

10 Women on HRT should have a check up every six months,

even if everything seems normal. Most doctors like to do a breast test, a blood pressure check and, maybe, an internal examination.

MIGRAINE

3 migraine control techniques to try

Migraine headaches are very common and affect three to four times as many women as men. They often affect teenagers and there is frequently a family history. The symptoms can be horrific and can affect a sufferer's whole life.

Pain is, of course, the worst and most significant symptom. It usually starts on one side of the head and is often accompanied by itching eyes, a stuffed up nose and a sensitivity to bright lights or loud noises.

Other symptoms can include a change in mood, temporary or partial blindness, chills, shaking and dizziness. Many patients feel sick and some actually are sick. Most sufferers have to lie down and rest for between 2 and 48 hours.

Exactly what causes migraine is still a mystery, though experts agree that stress is probably the most common trigger. When you are under pressure your body automatically increases the supply of blood to your muscles and reduces the supply of blood to your brain. Once the stressful moment is over the blood vessels to your brain suddenly open up again and blood surges through. It is this sudden flow of blood into the brain which is thought to cause the migraine headache.

This explains why migraine sufferers often notice that their headaches are worst just when they begin to relax—at the weekend for example.

Apart from resting and taking whatever pills your doctor has recommended there are several things you can do that may help you.

1   Try to avoid foods that may trigger an attack. Foods that are particularly likely to cause problems include cheese, chocolate, some types of wine—mainly red—and fruits such as

oranges and lemons. Some migraines are brought on by tobacco or alcohol. Next time you feel a migraine coming on try to write down everything you've eaten or done in the previous 24 hours. After a while you may be able to spot a pattern and see something that may be causing your headaches.

2   Learn to relax. Many migraine sufferers are perfectionists—they have to do everything just right. If something isn't perfect they worry. Someone once told me that a typical migraine sufferer is a woman who has to empty the ashtray as soon as someone has tapped ash into it.

3   There is a relatively new technique that may help you. Since migraines are associated with a narrowing and opening of the blood vessels the pain can sometimes be stopped by using a technique which deliberately stops the blood vessels from getting narrow in the first place. This technique depends on the fact that blood vessels supplying the brain are controlled in exactly the same was as blood vessels supplying the hands. Lie down and relax. Then close your eyes and imagine that your hands are getting warmer. It may help if you imagine that you are holding your hands in front of a fire. If you can do this successfully (and thousands can) then the blood vessels supplying your hands and brain will not narrow but will stay large to allow blood to flow into your hands to cool them! Once you have mastered this technique—which you will need to practise—you'll be able to use it whenever you feel a migraine coming on. Eight out of ten sufferers can help themselves this way.

MISCARRIAGE

Among younger women one in every five pregnancies ends in a miscarriage. The risks increase steadily with age and the incidence of miscarriages among forty-year-old women is double that of younger women.

When an egg and a sperm meet they do not always produce a perfect embryo and a miscarriage is nature's way of dealing with the problem. Less commonly a miscarriage may be caused becausea woman has an illness or a problem (such as fibroids) affecting her womb.

The first sign of a miscarriage is usually bleeding and the only remedy most doctors recommend is bed rest.

Once a woman has lost one baby there is no real increase in her likelihood of losing another. Only when a woman has lost two or more babies in early pregnancy is it accepted that she faces an increased risk of miscarriage.

After a miscarriage most doctors like women to wait at least three and preferably six months before getting pregnant again— to give their bodies a chance to recover properly. Most women who have miscarriages go on to have perfectly normal subsequent pregnancies, labours and babies.

After a miscarriage most women suffer a mixture of painful emotional responses—guilt and depression often being dominant. Women feel guilty because they fear that they may have lost their babies because of something they did (or did not do). There is usually no justification for this self criticism. The vast majority of miscarriages occur simply because the baby has not developed properly.

It is important that women who have lost babies should be encouraged to mourn fully so that their sadness can be put properly behind them.

MOUTH

☞ *See* Teeth.

MOUTH ULCERS

Mouth ulcers, also known as aphthous ulcers, can be found anywhere in the mouth (under your tongue, beneath your lower or upper lip or at the base of your gums are most common) and are incredibly sore.

There are lots of theories about how mouth ulcers develop, but two specific factors seem worth remembering.

First, physical trauma can often bring on an ulcer. If you slip with a toothbrush you may find an ulcer developing a few days later.

Second, stress and anxiety can make mouth ulcers more likely. If you're suddenly getting a lot of ulcers it may be because you're run down or you've been overdoing things.

There are lots of things that you can buy from the chemist but to be honest I've not much faith in any of them. Mouth ulcers should be gone in 7–10 days and the pain is usually at its worst for no more than a couple of days. If a mouth ulcer lasts longer than that or bleeds then you should see your doctor. You should also see him if you've never had one before and you're not sure what they look like.

MUMPS

Mumps is an infectious viral disease which is relatively uncommon under the age of 5.

The symptoms usually begin with a headache and a general feeling of not being well accompanied by various aches and pains. There may be a fever, too. Sometimes the first sign is a swelling which appears in front of one or both ears and possibly under the chin as well. The swelling is usually fairly noticeable and makes eating or talking painful.

Mumps is fairly infectious and symptoms will normally develop within three weeks of initial contact. The patient will be infectious from two days before the swelling appears until it has completely disappeared. Adults who have not had the disease should keep well away since mumps can be particularly painful if it attacks the testicles or ovaries.

NOSEBLEEDS

There are many causes of nosebleeds—including allergies, hay fever, infections, weak blood vessels and faults in the blood clotting mechanism—but bumps or punches on the nose are probably the commonest causes.

The majority of nosebleeds will stop by themselves whatever you do. That's why there are so many beautiful old myths about putting cold keys down the back of the victim's shirt or putting ice on his neck. These old fashioned tricks work for the simple reason that the nose bleeding would have probably stopped anyway.

To stop a nosebleed get the victim to lean forwards slightly, to breathe through his mouth and to squeeze his nose just below the bridge. Tell him not to speak, swallow, sniff or in any other way disturb the clotting blood. He must keep squeezing for between 5 and 10 minutes (the longer the better).

If this technique doesn't work and bleeding starts again when the squeezing stops, there may be a clot in the nose stopping the broken vessel from healing.

If you can't stop a nose bleed in 20 minutes ask your doctor for help. You should also ask for help if nosebleeds persist, recur or are accompanied by any other symptoms—or if they worry you!

OVERWEIGHT

18 tips to help you slim successfully

1   Try to set yourself easy slimming targets. If you try to get rid of all your unwanted weight in a month you will probably fail. Decide what your ideal weight should be and then aim at losing two pounds a week.

2   Remember that regular exercise will help to tone up your muscles *and* burn up a few extra calories. You don't have to do anything you don't enjoy. Two of the best—and most stress-free—exercises are swimming and walking.

3   Try to resist the temptation to weigh yourself every day. Weigh yourself once a week.

4   Don't let other people decide what you eat (or when you eat it). If you're full—stand up for yourself and say so!

5   Remember Coleman's First Golden Rule of Slimming: Only ever eat when you are hungry. Coleman's Second

Golden Rule of Slimming is: Stop when you are full. Every time you are about to put food into your mouth ask yourself whether or not you really *need* it.

6   Whenever you feel hungry and you find yourself reaching for food wait five minutes. Then—if you *still* feel hungry—you can eat.

7   Try not to put sugar in drinks.

8   Make a real effort to eat most of your meals sitting at the table rather than slumped in front of the television. You need to concentrate on what you are doing if you are going to use the power of your mind to help you slim successfully.

9   Never be afraid to throw food away if you don't want it. Don't eat up scraps just so that they 'won't be wasted'.

10 Try not to worry about weighing food or counting calories— that can be really boring. Learn to let your body help you diet by deciding when—and how much—you need to eat.

11 When you sit down to a meal sit for a moment or two and relax. Try to get rid of accumulated tensions. Then—and only then—start to eat. And eat slowly. If you concentrate on what you are doing you will be far more likely to hear your body 'talking' to you and telling you when you are 'full'.

12 Acquire a new habit. Try stopping between courses for a short rest. If you've had enough to eat get up and leave the table. If you stay sitting at the table after you've finished eating there is a risk that you will nibble at whatever is left.

13 Learn not to eat in the evening. If you eat when you're about to go to bed your body will store the unwanted calories as fat. Do most of your eating early in the day—so that your body can burn up the calories.

14 Whenever you have to have a big meal try to have a snack half an hour beforehand. The snack will *spoil* your appetite and ensure that you feel full long before you do your diet too much damage.

15 Make sure that you never reward yourself with food. If you want to celebrate do so with a bunch of flowers, a new tape

or a book or magazine.

16 Put a little time in trying to work out *how* you acquired *your* bad eating habits. What bad eating habits did you learn as a child? Awareness of your bad eating habits will make them easier to conquer.

17 Many people who find slimming alone difficult benefit by joining a slimming club. There are hundreds of slimming clubs around. Look in the local telephone book or ask your doctor. Many people get support and encouragement from slimming with others.

18 Try to give up eating 'main' meals. If you eat five or six small snacks instead of three large meals a day you will help your body adjust its calorie intake to its needs. People who 'snack' lose weight much more successfully than people who over–fill themselves with food three or four times a day.

OVERWEIGHT CHILDREN

10 ways to keep your child slim

A lifetime of obesity and dieting often begins in childhood.

Children who are fat often stay fat—and find it extremely difficult to lose excess weight later in life.

Here are some tips to help you try to stop your child becoming overweight:

1 Breast fed babies are probably less likely to become fat than bottle fed babies.

2 Wait until your baby is at least 6 months old before introducing solids.

3 Don't force your child to empty his bottle or clear his plate if he has had enough to eat. And remember to give him slightly less food next time.

4 Don't use food as a punishment or a reward. If you do then your child will associate food with emotional as well as physical needs.

5 Make sure that your child has a good breakfast but eats as

little as possible in the evening when the body's calorie requirements are at their lowest.

6 Encourage your child to eat when he is hungry as far as possible. Do not allow children to read or watch television when they are eating. The child who eats while doing something else will not be aware of his appetite control centre. He will just keep cramming food into his mouth automatically, regardless of whether or not he is still hungry.

7 Try to keep your child out of the habit of eating lots of sweets. Sweets ruin the teeth and are usually rich in calories. Teach your child to understand which foods are fattening.

8 Encourage your child to take regular exercise. Too many parents insist on carrying their children everywhere by motor car.

9 Keep a check on your child's weight. If he or she seems to be gaining weight too quickly then try to correct this. It will be easier to make a modest correction now than to try to deal with a massive weight problem in a year or two's time.

10 If you are overweight then you too should try to control your weight. Your children will find weight control difficult to understand if they see their parents eating anything and everything—and ignoring their own weight problem.

PARENTS

How to be a good one

If you want to take on a job that involves real responsibility, you will usually have to undergo a period of training.

If you want to drive a bus you will have to pass a test and get a special licence. If you want to become a policeman or a nurse or train driver you will have to study and pass exams before you will be allowed to take responsibility for the lives of others.

But there is one *very* responsible job for which absolutely no training is required—and for which very little training or advice is ever provided or made available: parenthood.

It has been well known now for many years that the way

parents bring up their children has a tremendous influence on how those children behave and live their lives.

Here are ten basic rules which are straightforward and easy to follow.

1   DON'T PUSH TOO HARD

We live in a competitive society and children of all ages are encouraged to do well. Do take care not to turn the screw too tight. Children commonly suffer from stress because they are trying too hard to please their parents.

Remember that stress induced tummy ache is far commoner than appendicitis in children. And it is not unknown for children under 10 to develop ulcers. Don't put too much pressure on children to do well on the sports field either. I have seen toddlers crying because their football team has been beaten. And I've met children with hands blistered by hours of practice with the tennis racquet or golf club.

2   GIVE YOUR CHILD RULES

Children desperately need rules. They need boundaries. They need to know how far they can go. If you don't give a child boundaries then he will push and push and push to see just how far he can go. He will do this not because he wants to be naughty but because he *needs* to know what he can and cannot do. You do not have to make up all the rules in advance, of course. Make them up as they are needed, and explain them. But once you have made up rules then you must ensure that they are kept to.

3   BE CONSISTENT

It is vital that you are consistent. If dad tells a 12-year-old that she has to be home by 10.30 pm and mum tells her that she can stay out all night then she child will inevitably become confused. She will lose respect for her parents. She will use the inconsistency. But she will also be alarmed and frustrated by it.

If mum tells a 5-year-old that he cannot play football in the garden but dad says he can, the child will be mixed up. He won't know where he stands and he'll be unhappy.

Parents should also remain consistent from one week to another. Nothing confuses children more than finding the rules changing each week. And they should apply the same rules to all their children. Children can accept that other kids from other families may have to follow different rules. But when different rules are applied to kids in the same family then the result is anger and bitterness.

4   DON'T MAKE YOUR CHILDREN GROW UP TOO SOON

Many children who are struggling to cope with the physical, mental and emotional problems of childhood or puberty are also expected to deal with adult responsibilities. Growing up is not easy. Don't try to speed things up. And try to let your child enjoy his childhood. He won't get another one.

5   PICK YOUR PUNISHMENTS CAREFULLY

I don't believe that parents should beat their children. But occasionally a smack can help. A light smack on the back of the legs or bottom smarts a little but shouldn't cause any physical damage. Alternatively, punish a child by depriving him of a TV programme he likes. The important thing about a punishment is that it should be appropriate, fair, consistent and, most important of all, short lived. If you keep a punishment going for days or even weeks then you will create more problems.

6   NEVER MANIPULATE YOUR CHILDREN

Parents often manipulate their children by saying things like: 'You wouldn't do that if you loved me'. Emotional blackmail of this kind can do long lasting damage to a sensitive child. A quick smack will do far more good and far less harm than subtle, psychological blackmail.

7   PROTECT YOUR CHILD AGAINST NASTY INFLUENCES

There is no 'proof' that violent TV programmes make children grow up to be violent. But the circumstantial evidence is overwhelming. I believe that TV violence causes far more problems than TV nudity or sex shows. Ban video nasties from your home and switch off when violent cop shows come on.

8   LET YOUR CHILDREN REBEL

Children need to rebel against their parents. It is part of growing up. Let your children know if you disapprove of something they are doing. But don't ban it unless you feel that a ban is really necessary. If your daughter dresses in bizarre clothes and you say nothing she will be disappointed. She expects disapproval. She wants you to notice. She needs you to moan at her. But don't insist that she dresses in a nice frock all the time. Rebelling is a natural, healthy, essential part of growing up.

9   DON'T SPOIL YOUR CHILDREN

Teach your children the value of hard work. Teach them to earn special treats and pocket money by performing small chores.

10   GIVE DAILY HUGS, CUDDLES AND KISSES

The most important rule of my ten. Don't forget to hug, cuddle and kiss your kids every day. And tell them that you love them at least once a day too.

PHOBIAS

Phobias—irrational, intense and uncontrollable fears—seem to be on the increase. They often start in childhood and frequently lead to panic attacks. Eight out of ten sufferers are women.

The ten commonest phobias are:

1   A fear of leaving home
2   A fear of storms—including thunder and lightning
3   A fear of enclosed spaces such as lifts
4   A fear of spiders
5   A fear of death and dying
6   A fear of dogs or cats
7   A fear of flying
8   A fear of heights
9   A fear of the dark

10 A fear of dentists and doctors—but especially needles

Gentle 'deconditioning' is the most effective way you can help yourself deal with a phobia. If you're frightened of cats try learning as much as you can about them. Read a book about cats. Look at cat pictures. Look at cats from a distance. Only when you start to feel more at ease with cats should you try picking one up.

If you are afraid of leaving the house try going out in small stages. Walk down the garden path. Go round to a friend's home. Gradually increase the distance you travel. Get friends to come with you.

Many phobics can overcome their problems by themselves. But if you need help talk to your doctor—he will be able to refer you to an expert.

PILES

☞ *See* Haemorrhoids.

PNEUMONIA

Pneumonia is an infection—and inflammation—of the lungs which can be caused by a wide variety of different bacteria, viruses and other organisms; it kills far more women than men and mostly affects the very old and the very young. Individuals such as alcoholics who have reduced immunity to infection are especially at risk.

The initial symptoms include: high temperature, shortness of breath, shivering, sweating, and a cough that produces nasty coloured sputum.

Penicillin and other antibiotics can often—but not always—cure infections.

To reduce your risk of contracting pneumonia:

- Eat a healthy diet—containing plenty of fresh fruit and vegetables.
- Keep your lungs healthy by avoiding breathing in too much smoky or dirty air.

- Avoid people who smoke.
- Help keep your immune system strong by making sure that you don't drink too much alcohol!

POISONING

10 ways to avoid it happening

Every year thousands of people are poisoned—especially children. Many die and many more suffer agonies. Poisoning is rarely really accidental and here are some basic guidelines to follow.

1   Child–resistant containers may be a nuisance but they do act as an effective deterrent. If you have children in the house always ask for medicines with child–proof lids.

2   Keep all medicines, even those you buy over the counter, in a special, locked cabinet well out of harm's way.

3   When a child visits an older relative make sure that there are no pills or medicines left lying around.

4   Never put poisons (household cleaners, garden products etc.) into containers other than those in which they came.

5   Teach your children the dangers of household products.

6   Throw away any unwanted medicines or chemicals—but don't simply put them in the dustbin: take them to your local chemist for disposal.

7   Never encourage children to take medicines by pretending they are sweets or saying that they taste nice.

8   Keep all household cleaners and other dangerous products locked away.

9   If you are working with a poisonous substance never leave it unattended—even for a few seconds.

10 Never remove labels from containers containing poisons.

If you suspect that someone has taken a poison act quickly—it is an emergency. Either call for medical help or take the patient direct to a hospital.

PREGNANCY

20 things every woman should know

1   Pregnancy is not an illness. You may fall ill while you are pregnant just as you may fall ill when you are cooking Sunday lunch, getting married or making love. But that inevitable risk doesn't make pregnancy itself an illness. Most women need no treatment during pregnancy and only need regular check ups to make sure that everything is going according to plan. Urine tests are done to test for sugar and protein and infection. Blood samples are taken to test for blood group and anaemia. Blood pressure is checked regularly.

2   Although a missed period is usually regarded as the classic sign of pregnancy other tell–tale symptoms include: feeling sick in the morning; breasts tingling and becoming bigger; needing to pass urine more often than usual; vaginal discharge; feeling tired; going off things like coffee, tobacco and fatty food. Some women just *feel* pregnant. Pregnancy tests work by detecting a hormone in the urine and are usually only reliable a month after conception.

3   Pregnancy usually lasts 40 weeks, counted from the first day of the last menstrual period. For the first eight weeks of pregnancy the developing baby is known as an 'embryo'. After that it is known as a 'foetus'.

4   The average mother-to-be will put on 28 pounds (12.7 kg) during her pregnancy—three quarters of it during the last 20 weeks. The average baby weighs seven and a half pounds (3.4 kg) and the placenta weighs another three pounds (1.4 kg). The remaining weight gain is increased fat stores and retained water. Within six weeks of giving birth most women get back to their original weight.

5   An increased appetite is normal. Many pregnant women have cravings for particular foods. Small, frequent meals are best. Don't fill up on 'stodgy' foods but try to eat plenty of fresh fruit, vegetables and high fibre foods.

6   Pregnant women should not smoke or drink alcohol. A woman who smokes will probably give birth to a baby who is lighter than he should be. The baby may be born premature and there is a greater risk of complications. There is a greater risk that a woman will lose her baby if she drinks booze while pregnant. And there is a greater risk that the baby will be born with an abnormality of some kind. There aren't any safe limits. The only way to reduce the risk to zero is not to smoke or drink alcohol at all.

7   A growing number of women have their babies at home. Some surveys show that there are greater risks in having a baby at home and some show that the risks are greater in hospital. Many women who have their babies at home enjoy the experience more. And the risk of infection is lower away from the hospital. But there is no doubt that if something goes wrong the risks will be greater in a bedroom than they will be in a special hospital unit. A few years ago women used to spend a week in hospital to have a baby. These days most women have short stay confinements and are in and out quickly.

8   Over 80% of women around the world give birth sitting, standing or squatting—with gravity helping. Giving birth lying down is a fashion that was created by a French king who wanted to see his mistress give birth but wanted it all happening at a convenient height for him. Talk to your doctor and midwife in advance about the best position for you.

9   Pregnant women should talk over with their partners the question of whether or not *he* should be in the delivery room. There are no rules. Some men prefer to pace up and down outside. And some women prefer their men to keep well out of the way. This is a decision you should take together.

10 Many women continue to enjoy sex throughout pregnancy—though choosing the right position is vital. The 'woman on top' positions are usually better than the 'missionary' position. Pregnant women should avoid: sex

while bleeding, violent sex, and sex if there is a risk of miscarriage. These days the rules are relaxed. Some women enjoy intercourse right up until the end of their pregnancies. Ask your doctor if it is safe for *you*. If you get the go ahead then just find a position that is comfortable for you both.

11 Three quarters of pregnant women work right up to the last month of their pregnancy. Women who have office work can obviously work longer than women whose jobs entail heavy physical work.

12 Breast milk is the best food your baby can get. It is perfectly formulated *and* it contains special substances which will help provide protection against infection. There are also psychological advantages to breast feeding since many women find it helps them to develop a close relationship with their baby.

13 A growing baby is most vulnerable to damage during its first three months. Apart from tobacco and alcohol drugs of many kinds can cause problems. No pregnant woman should take any drug (including medicines bought over the counter from the chemist) without first checking with her doctor.

14 About 1 in 80 mothers–to–be give birth to more than one baby. Twins, triplets etc. are commoner in pregnant women who are over thirty years old. Twins and other multiple pregnancies are more likely to be born premature.

15 Food passes through the intestines more slowly during pregnancy (so that more nutrients can be absorbed for the growing baby) so constipation is common among pregnant women. Fresh fruit and vegetables and plenty of fluids and fibre will help cure the problem naturally.

16 During pregnancy hormone levels vary. An increase in the amount of circulating oestrogen helps stimulate the uterus, increase the size of the nipples, boost the development of the breasts and increase the quantity of vaginal secretions. It also increases the production of body building protein and relaxes ligaments and joints ready for the delivery of the baby. The increase in progesterone increases breathing rate

and body temperature and controls the muscles. Other hormones help the breasts to grow, increase energy production and darken the nipples.

17 Many pregnant women suffer from backache (can be helped by wearing flat shoes and resting frequently); varicose veins (can be helped by wearing elastic stockings); swollen feet (can be helped by resting in the afternoons with the feet higher than the body); nausea (can be helped by eating small meals); breast tenderness (can be helped by wearing a bra that provides plenty of support).

18 Nine out of ten pregnant women develop stretch marks on their abdomens or breasts. There are many creams available but a massage with a plain moisturising cream will probably be as useful as anything else. A good, supporting bra will reduce the risk of stretch marks developing on the breasts. Stretch marks usually fade afterwards.

19 Most pregnant women feel their baby beginning to move by the 20th week of pregnancy.

20 Pregnant women often find that their moods are changeable. They may feel tearful, irritable or depressed for no obvious reason. This is usually due to hormone changes. But some women feel a sense of real and rare contentment during pregnancy!

PRE-MENSTRUAL SYNDROME

5 tips

Fifty per cent of all women suffer uncomfortable, painful and annoying symptoms before their periods. The symptoms vary but include: tension, irritability, depression, headaches, indigestion, diarrhoea, constipation, breast tenderness, swollen ankles, palpitations, faintness, dizziness, susceptibility to heat or cold, sleeplessness and changes in sexual interest.

If you suffer from any of these symptoms before your periods:

1   Go and see your doctor. If your doctor can't help you, ask him to arrange an appointment with a gynaecologist.

2   If you suffer from tender breasts or swollen ankles avoid salt, coffee, tea and alcohol before your periods.

3   Eat regular meals to help keep your blood sugar level steady.

4   Lose any excess weight—it may help.

5   Talk to your partner. His understanding your problem won't make it go away—but it will make it easier to bear.

PROSTATE GLAND

Facts all men should know

There are three common conditions which affect the prostate gland: first, enlargement; second, prostatitis, an inflammation of the prostate gland which unlike the other two common prostate problems often affects men under 35; and third, cancer of the prostate gland—an extremely common cancerous condition among men. Any man who suspects that he could have any of these disorders should, of course, see his doctor straight away.

1   ENLARGED PROSTATE GLAND

One in three men over 50 and one in two men over 60 have an enlarged prostate gland. Half of all these individuals show symptoms. An enlargement of the prostate gland may be benign or malignant.

There are several possible reasons why a prostate gland may enlarge. First, not responding to a need to pass urine seems likely to cause problems. Men who sit for long periods and can't go to the toilet—taxi drivers, bus drivers, airline pilots and so on—are likely to end up in difficulty. Second, heavy sexual stimulation without relief may lead to problems. Sexual petting or stimulation which doesn't lead to ejaculation within a decent period—and which keeps the prostate gland working too hard and too long without doing anything—seems likely to cause problems. It is possible that a man who thinks about sex a lot without ejaculating may be putting pressure on his prostate gland. Other factors which seem likely to increase the risk of prostatic obstruction include stress, smoking, cold, damp weather, drinking too much alcohol and some drugs.

The symptoms of an enlarged prostate gland include painful urination, frequent urination—particularly at night—and an inability to empty the bladder properly. Sufferers may also notice that their stream is more of a dribble and that they have difficulty in starting a stream of urine. An enlarged prostate gland may also lead to impotence, premature ejaculation and low back pain. The urine may be a strange colour too.

If the prostate gland becomes very enlarged then it may be necessary to remove part of it surgically.

To try to avoid getting an enlarged prostate you should keep fit, keep sexually active—and that includes masturbation if necessary—avoid too much alcohol and avoid unnecessary drugs.

2 PROSTATITIS

Prostatitis is an inflammation of the prostate gland—it may also lead to an inflammation of the urethra (the tube which carries urine from the bladder). This condition is fairly common among men under 35 and can be triggered by a sexually transmitted disease or by any infection brought from another part of the body—for example, an infection from the tonsils, the sinuses or the teeth. The disorder seems more likely among men who aren't sexually active. To minimise the risk of developing the condition it is wise to drink plenty of fluid—preferably water—in order to maintain a good flow of urine.

If acute prostatitis isn't treated then it can develop into chronic prostatitis—causing a blockage which may need surgery.

In mild cases the symptoms can include passing urine more often than usual, mostly at night; a slight fever; and an inability to empty the bladder properly. In more severe cases there may be a pain in the area between the scrotum and the anus.

The treatment will depend on the symptoms. If the pain is severe then the patient may need to go to bed. An antibiotic may be needed to treat the infection. Plenty of fluids may help but alcohol should be avoided.

3 CANCER OF THE PROSTATE

Cancer of the prostate is a disorder which is responsible for a large number of male deaths every year: 80% of cases of cancer of the prostate occur in men who are over 65 years of age.

The symptoms of prostate cancer may well be similar to those of a benign or harmless enlarged gland—although it is possible to have prostate cancer with few or maybe even no symptoms. The symptoms will depend on just where in the gland the cancer is. Common signs include a poor urinary stream, increased frequency, diminished urinary stream and an incomplete emptying of the bladder. Impotence occurs sometimes and there may be blood in the urine.

A diagnosis is usually made by a finger examination in the rectum, by X-rays and by a biopsy of the gland—blood tests also help. If the enlargement is cancerous then the prostate is usually removed surgically. In addition drugs may be needed and some men may be helped by having their testes removed. Cancer of the prostate is primarily—but not exclusively—a disorder affecting the elderly. Many sufferers survive for quite a while after the disease is first diagnosed—and many die of other consequences of old age.

PUBERTY

Puberty, the time when boys turn into men and girls turn into women, usually starts at the age of about ten in girls and about twelve in boys—continuing to the ages of 16 and 18 respectively. The onset of puberty is influenced by many factors including race, genetics and nutrition. If a girl has not shown any signs of puberty (breast development, pubic hair, growth spurt and the onset of menstruation) by the age of thirteen then medical advice should be sought, though in most cases there will be no underlying problem and puberty will eventually arrive. Most boys show signs of early puberty (pubic hair, larger penis, growth spurt, facial hair, voice breaking) by the age of fifteen.

RASHES

Some rashes are infectious while others are not. Some rashes are itchy. Others are quite insignificant and go away by themselves. There are blotchy rashes, spotty rashes, lumpy rashes and blistery rashes. There are infected rashes, allergy rashes and rashes that no one (not even the experts) can explain.

Many rashes are made worse because they are left too long without treatment. Other rashes become very bad because they are treated the wrong way.

Here are three basic rules about rashes that are well worth remembering:

1   If you don't know the exact cause of a rash—and the correct treatment—don't try treating it yourself.

2   If a rash gets worse while being treated then there is a good chance that the treatment is making the rash worse.

3   If a rash doesn't disappear, continues to spread or is accompanied by other symptoms—get medical advice.

1   HEAT RASH

This is probably the commonest type of rash to affect babies and young children. Although the heat rash usually occurs in warm weather it *can* occur in the cold if the child is overdressed. Heat rashes usually begin on the cheeks, shoulders, skin creases and bottom. The rash consists of tiny red spots the size of a pin head. Blond or red headed children are most likely to suffer. The first thing to do is to cool the sufferer. If the outside temperature is high then sponging with tepid water may help, but otherwise remove some clothes. Keep your patient cool and sprinkle a little powder on the rash. It is important to remember that detergents and bubble baths may make heat rashes worse.

2   NAPPY RASH

Nappy rashes are pretty common too. They tend to be red, rough and rather scaly, and confined to the area of skin covered by the nappy. A nappy rash may be caused by the detergent in which the nappy has been washed or it may be caused by contact of the skin with the urine. Once a nappy rash has developed it is important to expose the rash to the air as much as possible. Do ensure that if washable nappies are used they are really washed thoroughly and rinsed well. Change nappies frequently and avoid waterproof pants where you can. Disposable nappies are particularly useful—especially if a rash has already developed. Zinc and castor oil ointment may help if rubbed on the affected area.

3 ALLERGY RASHES

Allergy rashes tend to appear fairly suddenly. They are often widespread. They usually itch. When a medicine has been taken in the previous two weeks it is possible that the drug was the cause. Penicillin is a common culprit but any medicine can cause an allergy reaction. If you suspect that a medicine has caused a rash telephone your doctor straight away for advice. The doctor will have to decide whether or not to carry on with the treatment. The itching usually associated with a drug allergy rash can often be eased by the use of ordinary calamine lotion. If this doesn't work then your doctor may prescribe an antihistamine tablet or medicine. If you think that an allergy rash has been produced by something that your child has eaten or drunk you should consider anything eaten or drunk within the last month as a possible culprit.

4 INFECTIOUS RASHES

Differentiating between the causes of the types of rash that develop in children can be difficult. Chickenpox is usually easy to diagnose because although the infection starts with a red blotchy rash the spots quickly become watery blisters. The main problem is in differentiating between measles and rubella. The measles rash is usually blotchy whereas a rubella rash seems rather spottier. Another way of telling the difference is to see how the patient feels. A child with measles is almost always fairly poorly whereas a child with rubella will probably feel quite well. Of these three rashes only the chickenpox rash usually itches and the best treatment is probably calamine lotion.

RAYNAUD'S DISEASE

The majority of sufferers of Raynaud's disease are women between the ages of 12 and 40. The condition is common among adults but extremely rare among children.

The usual symptoms are cold, dead, white and painful fingers (though the toes can be affected too) and the problem usually develops in the cold weather when the small arteries which normally provide blood to the hands and feet shut down and go into spasm. As the blood flow returns, the fingers and toes gradually turn from white to blue and then, eventually, to red. During an attack the fingers may feel numb and may burn. As the blood flows back into the tissue there is frequently a tingling feeling. The lack of an adequate blood supply may lead to infections and ulcers.

The cause of Raynaud's disease seems to be an extreme sensitivity to cold—possibly due to a malfunctioning autoimmune system—although stress is another known factor. Tobacco—which constricts the arteries—often triggers the disease which is relatively rare among non smokers.

The usual advice to sufferers is to wear warm gloves and socks in order to keep the hands and feet warm but this really isn't enough. Because the blood vessels automatically shut down (in order to preserve heat) when the body is cold sufferers need to keep their entire bodies warm all the time.

Sufferers are always warned to wear gloves when using the fridge or freezer since the impact of the intense cold can shut down the arteries for long periods.

Raynaud's disease is considered incurable at the moment but there are ways to make symptoms less painful:

- Moving to a warmer climate is, for many, impractical but Raynaud's does seem less common in hot countries.
- Avoiding stress helps.
- An occasional glass of alcohol may help by opening up the blood vessels.
- Biofeedback training in which sufferers are taught how to use the power of their minds to expand the size of their

blood vessels is one of the most promising techniques.

Raynaud's disease usually gets gradually worse over the years. In severe cases doctors may be able to help.

In addition to Raynaud's disease there is also a condition known as Raynaud's phenomenon in which the same thing happens—but for an identifiable reason.

In Raynaud's phenomenon the arteries are sent into spasm either by an underlying disease or as a side effect of the use of one of a number of different prescription drugs.

Relaxation

How to relax your body and your mind

Tension tightens your muscles because your body is responding to the stress you're under. Your body assumes that because you feel anxious you are in danger. It assumes that you are physically threatened and it tenses your muscles so that you will be better able to fight or run away.

But, of course, tensed muscles lead to headache, back pains and scores of other painful physical symptoms.

If you are going to learn how to conquer the stress in your life—and relax effectively—you *must* plan your relaxation programme carefully.

- If you've got children get someone else to look after them.
- If you've got a telephone take it off the hook.
- Go into a room where you can be quiet and alone.
- Close the curtains.
- Turn off the lights.
- Lie or sit down somewhere really comfortable.
- Close your eyes.

Now, follow my 20 point relaxation plan.

1   Clench your right hand as tightly as you can, making a fist with your fingers. Count up to ten while you hold your fingers tight and tense. If you now gradually let your fingers unfold you will feel your muscles slowly relaxing.

2   Bend your right arm and try to make your right biceps

muscle stand out. Again, count up to ten. Then lay your arm down loosely by your side.

3 Relax your left hand in the same way that you relaxed your right hand.

4 Relax your right arm, then lay it down by your side and forget about it.

5 Curl the toes in your right foot as tightly as you can. Count up to ten. Then relax those muscles.

6 Move your right foot so that your toes are pointing up towards your knee. Count up to ten. You should feel the muscles in your calf becoming tighter. Then relax.

7 Try to push your right foot away from you. You should feel the muscles in your right thigh tightening up. Count up to ten. Then relax.

8 Relax your left foot.

9 Relax your left lower leg.

10 Relax your left thigh.

11 Tighten up the muscles in your bottom so that your whole body lifts up an inch or so. Count up to ten. Then relax.

12 Try to pull your abdominal muscles in towards your spine. Count up to ten. Then relax.

13 Take a big breath in. Count up to ten. Then relax.

14 Keep your head still and try to touch your ears with your shoulders. It will be impossible but try anyway. Count to ten. Then relax.

15 Stretch your neck as far away from your chest as you can. Count to ten. Then deliberately relax those muscles too. Move your head around in all directions to make sure that your neck muscles are free and easy.

16 Stretch the muscles of your back. Try to make yourself as tall as you can. Count to ten. Then relax.

17 Move your eyebrows as high as you can. Hold them high up while you count up to ten. Then relax.

18 Screw up your eyes very tightly. Pretend that someone is

trying to force them open. Count to ten; then, keeping your eyes closed, relax those muscles too.

19 Push your tongue out as far as it will go. Count to ten. Then relax.

20 Smile as wide as you possibly can. Count to ten. Then relax.

All this should have taken you slightly less than ten minutes. And every muscle in your body should now be thoroughly relaxed. Now you need to relax your *mind*.

Try to imagine that you are lying on a warm, sunny beach.

It is *your* personal, private beach. There is no one else there. And no one else will ever be allowed onto it.

Then use all your senses to help soothe away all your anxieties and all your everyday pressures.

● FEEL the sun on your face and body.

● LISTEN to the sound of the sea in the distance *and* the sound of seagulls circling high overhead.

● SMELL the salt sea air.

The more you can convince yourself that you are lying, relaxed and calm, on a warm, sunny beach the more effectively you will be able to escape from your daily worries.

If you practise this simple exercise *every day for a fortnight* you will find that you will gradually get more and skilled at relaxing your body and your mind.

Soon, you should be able to relax yourself within a minute.

And, most important of all, you will be able to relax wherever you are and whatever you are doing.

Within a fortnight you should be able to relax both your body and your mind: in a queue in your local shop, while waiting for a bus or train or while doing the washing up.

All you will have to do is to close your eyes and imagine that you are lying on your own, personal, warm, sunny beach.

RESTLESS LEGS SYNDROME

Many women complain that while they lie in bed at night their legs twitch. This is called the 'restless legs syndrome'.

It is one of the oldest of all disorders and was first described over 300 years ago. Caffeine is believed to be one of the major causes today. To avoid the problem try drinking less—or weaker—coffee or tea.

If you spend much of your time sitting down then mild exercise will probably help.

ROSACEA

The cause of rosacea, a long term skin problem in which the cheeks and nose are unusually red, is not known. The condition is commonest among women in their thirties, forties and fifties. In some cases the nose may also become bulbous and red. Drinking alcohol or a hot drink or even entering a hot room can trigger a temporary flushing of the skin on the face. It is possible that the disorder can be triggered in some cases by corticosteroid creams used to treat skin conditions. Some foods—notably coffee, tea, chocolate and spicy foods—may trigger the condition.

The temporary redness of early rosacea can sometimes develop into a permanent redness of the skin. The redness may sometimes be accompanied by spots which may look rather like acne.

The treatment of rosacea may involve the long term use of the drug tetracycline—but although this may suppress the symptoms it will not cure the problem. Rosacea sometimes disappears after a few years.

RUBELLA (GERMAN MEASLES)

Rubella (also sometimes known as german measles) is a very common infectious disease caused by a virus. The initial symptoms are usually those of a cold and possibly a tenderness behind the ears and at the back of the neck. The typical rash of german measles starts behind the ears and on the face and then spreads all over the body. The rash begins as small, flat pink spots but these later clump together to form red patches. There may be some itching but there isn't usually any fever.

The disease is fairly infectious and it may take three weeks for symptoms to develop. The patient is infectious from day one—before the appearance of the rash—until two days after it has gone.

There is no cure and there is not usually any need for specific treatment. There is, however, a vaccine available to protect against the disease. All girls approaching puberty should be vaccinated because of the risks associated with the disease during pregnancy. For this reason anyone who has german measles should be kept away from pregnant women.

If a pregnant women does catch german measles she may have a miscarriage or give birth to a deformed baby. The first three months of pregnancy are the most dangerous.

Other than the risks during pregnancy complications with german measles are rare but problems to watch out for include vomiting, ear ache and headache. These or any other unexpected symptoms warrant a visit from the doctor. Don't take anyone to a doctor's surgery if you think they could have rubella.

SCABIES

Scabies can affect the cleanest of families. It is very infectious and can be transmitted directly from one person to another or it can be passed on in infected clothing or bedding. It can live in discarded clothes or bedding for up to a week. It is commonly passed on from one individual to another when they are sharing a bed but outbreaks also occur in schools, hospitals and institutions of all kinds. The incubation period between initial contact and the development of symptoms—the itchy rash—is usually around six weeks.

If you look closely at the patient's skin you will probably be able to see the small, lined tracks leading from the blisters which show the direction in which the mites (called sarcoptes scabiei) have gone. The rash can appear anywhere on the body but is usually most noticeable on the hands and forearms and around the waist.

A special anti scabies skin remedy should be applied—obtainable from any doctor or pharmacist.

SCHOOL PHOBIA

School phobia will cause a child to show genuine physical signs of anxiety. When faced with the prospect of attending school he may breathe more quickly, sweat, feel nauseous or complain of 'butterflies' in his stomach. He may even faint.

The phobic child will do almost anything to avoid going to school. He may lie if necessary. He may be unable to live a normal life.

If you think your child may have school phobia then clearly you have to discover what is at the root of his phobia. It will normally be caused by something quite specific such as a fear of being bullied, fear of a particular teacher or teachers, fear of failure or fear of ridicule—it may, of course, be a combination of several of these factors.

Talking to the child and his teachers is the first step to resolving the problem. Give the child plenty of love, support and encouragement and if the problem persists ask your doctor if he can refer you and your child to a child psychologist.

SINUSITIS

The sinuses are cavities in the bones around the nose. They are usually filled with air. If the membranous lining of the facial sinuses becomes inflamed by infection the symptoms of sinusitis—pain, fever and a stuffy nose—may develop.

Antibiotics are usually prescribed to clear up the infection. Old fashioned steam inhalations often help a great deal by moistening the secretions within the sinuses.

Sleeplessness (Insomnia)

17 tips for people who can't sleep

It is while you are asleep that your batteries are recharged. During the daytime millions of bits and pieces of information are fed into your brain. Sleeping gives it its only real rest.

If you don't get the sleep you need then you will wake up tired, irritable, inefficient and depressed.

1   If you are kept awake by worry then you need to learn how to relax—and you may need to deal positively with some of the problems that are worrying you. Read the advice on Stress in this book.

2   If noise keeps you awake, try wearing ear plugs. You should be able to buy them quite cheaply at your local pharmacy.

3   If you are kept awake by pain, breathlessness—or any other symptoms—then tell your doctor and ask for treatment for the problem that is keeping you awake.

4   If you simply don't feel tired when you go to bed then maybe you are trying to get too much sleep. Some people only need five hours a night. Most of us need less sleep as we get older.

5   If you feel hungry at night then have a bite to eat before you go to bed. And remember that people who are slimming usually get less sleep than normal. If you are on a diet make sure that your late night nibble is a low calorie snack. Do not drink anything containing caffeine (e.g. tea or coffee) because caffeine will keep you awake. Try to avoid cigarettes: these are also a stimulant.

6   If your bed is uncomfortable, maybe you need a new one. Soggy or lumpy mattresses often keep people awake.

7   If you have recently been prescribed pills by your doctor ask him if the pills could be keeping you awake. And remember that if you have been taking tranquillisers or sleeping tablets for more than two weeks they can cause sleeplessness. But do *not* stop any pills without talking to your doctor.

8   If your bedroom is too stuffy and you cannot breathe at night improve the ventilation—e.g. by opening a window.

9   If your bed is cold invest in an electric blanket (but be sure to follow the manufacturer's instructions—and do not go to bed with the blanket on) or a hot water bottle.

10 If you have difficulty in turning off your mind when you get into bed then try reading a book before you go to sleep—preferably something not too demanding.

11 Have a brisk walk for 10–15 minutes or exercise in the house if you don't want to go outside. You will sleep better if you are physically tired rather than just mentally exhausted. If you try to go to bed directly after doing paperwork you will find that your brain won't stop buzzing: the things you have been thinking about will insist on popping into your mind.

12 Write down all your problems and worries in a notebook.

13 Warm the bed before you get into it. You will sleep better if you are warm. (If you use an electric blanket remember to turn it off before you get into bed).

14 Lie in a warm bath for 15 minutes before going to bed.

15 Go to bed with a relaxing book that you know you will enjoy. Don't go to bed with something that will make you think or worry.

16 When you are feeling tired close your eyes and take yourself off to somewhere relaxing, warm and beautiful.

17 If you do wake up or you do have difficulty in getting to sleep don't just lie there getting more and more uptight. Pick up your book and read another couple of chapters.

Sleeplessness in children

Few things worry parents more than having a child who does not sleep properly. However, if we classify something as 'normal' if it happens to more than half of the population then it is normal for a child to have a problem getting to sleep at some time or another.

Often there is some obvious reason for this.

If the television downstairs is on too loud or if the neighbours make a lot of noise then it will be hardly surprising if your child doesn't get to sleep. Similarly, children have difficulty in getting to sleep if the bedroom is too hot or too cold, if they are nervous or worried or frightened or if their bedroom is too stuffy.

It is sometimes said that babies do not sleep when they are teething. I think that is a myth—unless the teething is causing discomfort which is keeping the baby awake.

Children who are wet, hungry, in pain or short of breath will have difficulty in getting to sleep. A child who has been dozing on the couch all afternoon will be unlikely to fall asleep the minute he goes to bed.

Some young children manage to run the whole household around their disturbed and eccentric sleeping patterns. Some children won't go to sleep until they have been told a story. Others wont sleep unless they are allowed into bed with their parents. Others have to go through time consuming and wearisome rituals before they will even contemplate sleep. Often the sleeplessness is merely a bad habit and to solve the problem the parents must teach their child that he will not get any more attention until he learns to behave properly.

Try not to pay too much attention if your baby starts to cry at night when you are confident there is nothing wrong. Check that all is well but remember that if you get him out of bed to stop him crying you will have established a new bad habit.

And don't keep going into your child's bedroom to check that all is well. If you do that then your child will eventually get into the habit of lying awake waiting for your next visit.

The quickest way to deal with a child who has acquired bad habits and won't go off to sleep by himself unless he is told a story, brought into his parents' bedroom or allowed to go downstairs and have a drink and something to eat, is to avoid responding to his demands. You would have to do this for several nights to break the bad habit.

If you find this too harsh a prospect there is an alternative.

For the first week go into the bedroom and sit on his bed. Do not let him out of bed unless he has to go to the lavatory. For the second week go into the room, check that all is well and then leave. Don't sit on the bed at all. In the third week, open the door, check from the door that all is well and don't go into the room.

If you really want your child to acquire new sleeping patterns you will find that he will understand this—and a new habit will be formed.

SMOKING

How to give up

1   Make a list of all the places where you ever smoke (office, living room, bedroom, kitchen, car, train etc.). Put the list in order—with the place where you smoke most at the top. Now stop smoking at the place on the bottom of your list *today*. And each day work your way up your list—making a new place out of bounds.

2   Tell everyone you know that you are giving up smoking. Better still get them to sponsor you for your favourite charity. The longer you hold out the more money you collect—and the less likely you will be to start smoking again!

3   After getting your doctor's permission, take up very gentle exercise. When you realise how unfit smoking has made you then your incentive to give up will increase.

4   Put the money you save by *not* smoking into a special jar and use it to buy yourself something special. If you're a regular smoker you'll be surprised at how much you save.

5   Imagine the sort of situation where you are most likely to light up a cigarette. Now imagine yourself coping *without* smoking. Build up your self image and you won't need to smoke.

6   Buy a bead necklace or bracelet. When your fingers feel edgy without a cigarette between them keep them occupied

playing with your beads.

7   Quit smoking with a friend. Ring one another up when you feel you are weakening.

8   Don't do anything else difficult while you are giving up. Don't diet, don't take on extra responsibilities at work and don't tackle other personal or professional problems. You need all your mental strength to stop smoking.

9   Make yourself your favourite meals. Food will taste better when you stop smoking—take advantage of it.

10 Keep all your cigarette butts in a jar in front of you. The sight and smell will help reinforce your determination to stop.

Why giving up will improve your family's health

Children whose parents smoke are far more vulnerable to infections, far more likely to suffer from headaches, sickness and other common health problems than children whose parents do not smoke: they breathe in the secondhand cigarette smoke that is breathed out and it pollutes their lungs and damages their health.

Inevitably, children who are for ever ill and always losing time from school will drift behind in academic and sporting terms. They have a rotten start to life.

Here are two tips to help you stop smoking to help your child!

1   Put your nose an inch away from a full ashtray. Then take a deep breath. That is what you smell like to your child.

2   Buy your children (or the neighbour's children) water pistols. And tell them that they can 'shoot' you on sight every time they see you lighting up.

The evidence that 'passive' or secondhand smoking may be harmful

• At a world conference on lung health in Boston in 1990 it was estimated that passive smoking kills 50,000 Americans a year—two thirds of whom die of heart disease. That is, without a doubt, far, far more than the number of people who die from using *all* illegal drugs.

● According to the World Health Organization tobacco smoke in the environment is responsible for around one quarter of all the lung cancers which affect non smokers.

● A WHO. statement published in May 1991 warned that 'in marriages where one partner smokes and the other does not, the risk of lung cancer to the non smoker is 20–50% higher'.

● A report in Britain claimed that every year 17,000 children under the age of 5 are admitted to hospital because of tobacco smoke from their parents or people looking after them. The report, which reviewed 400 research papers, estimated that children whose parents smoke inhale the equivalent of 150 cigarettes a year. The same report also estimates that smoking by pregnant women causes 4,000 miscarriages of healthy babies each year.

● An American report concluded that women who breathe in other people's tobacco smoke are more likely to develop cervical cancer.

● Evidence presented at a scientific session of the American Heart Association showed that men who do not smoke are more likely to have heart disease if their partners smoke.

● Researchers in London have shown that smoking in the home can stunt children's growth.

● An Australian judge has branded the tobacco industry guilty of misleading and deceptive advertising in claiming that there is no scientific proof that passive smoking was a health risk. After a 90 day hearing the judge, who reviewed evidence from the United States, Europe and Australia, said the evidence showed that passive smoking caused respiratory diseases in young children, asthma and lung cancer.

● The United States Environmental Protection Agency concluded that passive smoking causes 3,800 lung cancer deaths each year in America.

● A scientist from the University of California has claimed that passive smoking ranks behind smoking and alcohol as the third leading preventable cause of death.

● Studies in Virginia, USA show that children of parents who smoke have an increased risk of heart disease.

Those are, I stress, just *some* of the research papers which show that passive smoking is dangerous. My advice is that you should keep your children clear of smokers as much as you can.

SNORING

5 tips to help you stop it

Snoring is no joke. Some snorers produce more noise than a pneumatic drill! One in three men snore regularly and half of all men snore occasionally. A third of all women snore occasionally too.

The sound of snoring is produced by the way air flows inside the nose and mouth. Any obstruction that gets in the way can produce snoring. Catarrh, polyps, nasal congestion, even ill fitting dentures can all cause snoring.

Here are some tips for conquering the problem:

1   If you're fat go on a diet. Thin people snore less.

2   Avoid alcohol or salty food late at night.

3   Exercise regularly—it does seem to help.

4   Most important of all try to sleep on your side rather than your back. Most snorers lie on their backs when they sleep.

5   If none of this works ask your doctor to arrange an appointment for you to see an Ear, Nose and Throat specialist. There may be an obstruction he can help you overcome.

SORE THROAT

☞ *See* Colds and flu.

SPRAINS

If the ligaments which hold together the two bone ends which make up a joint are pulled apart suddenly they may tear or stretch. That is a sprain. The ankle is the joint most likely to be sprained.

A sprained ankle will normally be swollen and painful. It will be difficult to move the joint without increasing the pain.

It is often difficult to differentiate between a sprain and a fracture and an X-ray will probably be needed. The usual treatment of a sprain is to put an ice pack on the joint, to wrap a compression bandage around the area and to raise the joint. Painkilling tablets may be needed. The joint should be rested.

SQUINT

The movement of each eye is controlled by a number of tiny muscles which are attached at one end to the eyeball and at the other end to the socket in which the eye sits. When the muscles aren't perfectly tuned the two eyes won't move together. The result is a squint. The type of squint will depend upon the position and duties of the affected muscle(s). Sometimes a squint is only obvious when the child looks in a particular direction.

Squints can occur at any age but appear most commonly during childhood. Some experts believe that between 5% and 8% of children have squints.

Squints can be corrected. But it is important to get advice as soon as you can. If a squint is left untreated a child may lose the sight in one eye.

STRESS

11 tips to help you conquer the stress in your life

Stress is the biggest killer of the twentieth century. It can damage your body and your mind and is a common cause of anxiety.

The symptoms of anxiety include shivering, sleeplessness, panic attacks, phobias and inability to relax. Many physical disorders—including heart disease, high blood pressure, asthma, indigestion, eczema, irritable bowel syndrome and alopecia—are caused by stress and anxiety.

The causes vary but include worry about work, money and relationships. Medical treatment often involves tranquillisers or sleeping tablets but it is now recognised that the drugs used can be addictive and may *cause* many problems of their own.

Here are ten tips for controlling the stress in your life.

1   Learn to recognise when you are under too much stress. Most of us have a weak point. Learn to recognise your weak point. It will tell you when you are under too much pressure.

The commonest early warning signs are:
- indigestion
- headaches
- diarrhoea
- sleeplessness
- palpitations
- tiredness
- wheezing
- irritability
- poor memory
- feeling tearful

If your doctor cannot find an explanation for any of these symptoms, they are probably a sign that you're under stress. Pull back a little. Do less. Take a break.

2   Cut out unnecessary stresses.

Make a list of all the things you are planning to do this week.

Now decide how much time you are going to spend on things *you* want to do. And how much on things that you are doing for *other* people.

Then see which list is longest.

Work out what your priorities are.

What can you cut from both lists?

3   Let your emotions show.

Do not be frightened to show that you are sad or angry.

Laugh when you feel happy.

Cry when you feel sad.

Bottling up your emotions leads to long term problems.

4   Organise your life.

By planning properly you will be able to reduce unexpected stresses.

5   Learn to value yourself.

Build yourself up by writing down all your virtues.

Look at the following list of words and underline the ones that apply to you:

careful, generous, kind, hard–working, creative, fair, thoughtful, attentive, honest, conscientious, tolerant, unselfish, friendly, considerate, good humoured, charitable, witty, wise, clever.

Make a list of all your other skills—and think of all the good things you can say about yourself.

6   Banish boredom from your life.

Try taking up a hobby that you find rewarding.

Or join a voluntary organisation that supports some cause you firmly believe in.

7   Learn to relax properly.

Imagine that you are lying on a grassy bank by a clear country stream.

Close your eyes.

Try to 'feel' yourself there.

Try to hear the water and the birds.

Try to feel the sunshine on your face. As you relax so your whole body—and your mind—will benefit.

8   Get rid of your worries by writing them down.

Get a piece of paper and a pencil.

Make a list of all the things that are worrying you.

Just writing them down will often help.

Now go through the list and decide exactly what you can do about each one.

9   Take your holidays.

Some people boast that they haven't had a holiday for years. That is crazy.

If you are uptight then you need to get away to relax.

Remember that short holidays taken often are probably more good to you than long, infrequent holidays taken when you are too exhausted to benefit.

10   Learn to do nothing.

Most of us are always in a rush.

Try to learn now how to do nothing occasionally.

11   Acquire a pet.

Everyone who has ever lived with a cat or dog will know that sharing your life with an animal can be soothing, calming and comforting. Now, at last, doctors have produced scientific evidence to support this belief. Patients suffering from anxiety, depression and stress related disorders such as high blood pressure have all been helped by learning to love animals.

●   Research in Australia which involved nearly 6,000 people showed that people who shared their lives with animals had lower blood pressure and lower cholesterol levels than people who didn't live with animals.

●   Research has shown that adults who live with dogs or cats suffer less from minor health problems such as colds, back ache and stomach problems.

●   Prisoners who are allowed contact with animals became less tense.

●   Patients in a psychiatric hospital who had failed to show any improvement when given drugs responded well when they were allowed to keep cats and dogs of their own.

Isolated individuals feel happier when they have an animal with whom they can share their lives. Lonely people benefit by having a dog or cat they can talk to. And people who wouldn't otherwise get enough exercise benefit because they go for walks!

Even fish in a tank can be therapeutic. American researchers have shown that hospital patients who watch fish in an aquarium are more relaxed than patients who don't.

There is, of course, a downside to all this. When a loved animal dies the grief can be just as real and the pain just as severe as when any other member of the family passes away. A survey of nearly 1,000 people who had recently lost loved animals showed that half became depressed and a quarter couldn't sleep.

It is important to remember this: people who have lost loved animals need just as much support and comfort as any other bereaved individual. (And don't just say: 'Get another one'. Would you say the same thing to someone whose spouse or parent has just died?)

Stress in children

Causes, consequences and solutions

You may think that stress is something that only affects adults. It isn't. Even for children life is full of stresses and strains which are so numerous and so varied that it is impossible to make a comprehensive list of them all. I have, however, produced a short list of some of the more common ways in which today's children are exposed to stress.

The causes of stress in children

1. THE PRESSURE TO SUCCEED

I don't think children have ever been put under quite as much pressure to succeed as they are these days. By the time they reach the age of six or seven children are already under a tremendous amount of pressure to do well at school. The pressure comes from both parents and teachers.

2. THE ACQUISITIVE SOCIETY

By the time they are old enough to vote your children will

have seen over 100,000 commercials on television—and countless thousand more in newspapers and magazines. In the cinema or listening to the radio your children will have been encouraged to believe that without buying this or that their lives cannot be complete. All this advertising inevitably causes frustration and anger.

3. THE PRESSURE TO MATURE

Too often children are forced to mature too soon. Parents don't allow their children to grow gently into maturity—they expect them to behave in a mature and sensible fashion right from the start. Youngsters who are deprived of their childhood—and forced to grow up too soon—will be more likely to suffer from stress.

4. TOO MUCH FEAR

Bad news surrounds us. Most adults worry about the world when they stop to think about what is going on. Children are the same. We cannot protect our children from all the bad news that fills the airwaves and newspapers. But we should take the time to talk about these things. Many children feel that they want to do something to try to stop violence and save the environment. Encourage them—for their sake as much as for the sake of society.

5. TOO MUCH GUILT

Parents put children under pressure in a lot of ways. Every time you say things like 'I bet J down the road doesn't treat his mother this way' you are putting your children under pressure and making them feel guilty. Simple phrases, often uttered without thought, can produce enormous stress.

The consequences of stress in childhood

Children react to stress in many different ways. Some children can cope with enormous stresses without developing signs or symptoms of illness. Others fall ill at the slightest stress. Some children complain of specific physical symptoms while others complain of rather vague symptoms such as tiredness.

Here are a few of the conditions which are known to be related to stress in children.

1. ABDOMINAL PAIN

When children complain of abdominal pain the first thing most parents and doctors think of is appendicitis. For many years doctors have, however, been puzzled by the fact that between a third and a half of all appendices which are removed in the operating theatre turn out to be perfectly healthy. In many cases no accurate diagnosis can be made when children complain of tummy aches. Now there is evidence to show that in many of these cases stress is the cause of the pain. Common as appendicitis is, it isn't as common a cause of abdominal pain in children as worry and anxiety.

When the pains are caused by stress they are usually situated in the centre of the abdomen, they are rather vague and they come and go. Stress induced abdominal pains can often be clearly related to a particular pressure. Tummy pains which stop a child going to school on a Monday morning are often a result of stress. Also, children can—and do—get indigestion. Over eating is the commonest cause. Eating green apples in large quantities can produce an indigestion type of pain. But worry and anxiety can cause indigestion too. Try to find out what the problem is if you think this is possible. It isn't unknown for children to get peptic ulcers as a result of worry and anxiety.

2. ACCIDENTS

Accidents are the commonest cause of death and serious injury in children over the age of one year. More children die of accidents than die of pneumonia, meningitis, cancer and heart disease put together. And yet most accidents aren't accidents at all. There is almost always a cause—and that cause is often stress. If your child is permanently decorated with bits of sticking plaster and bandage, you should ask yourself whether he might be under too much stress at home or at school. The child who is too anxious and under stress will fail to concentrate on what he is doing. He will be accident prone.

3. ANOREXIA NERVOSA

When children stop eating it is often because they are unable to cope with the pressures put on them by their parents. The girl who refuses to put on weight may be refusing to grow up and accept the accompanying responsibilities.

4. ASTHMA

Most children who have asthma are worse when they are under pressure. Indeed, there are some asthma sufferers who only suffer when they are under stress. Parents who openly row with one another or who put great pressure on their children may find that their children suffer from asthma which is difficult to treat. And parents who make too much fuss about a child's asthma may make things worse by making the child worry too.

5. BED WETTING

When children continue to wet their beds after the age of five or six years and doctors have excluded all the possible causes then the answer may be that the bed wetting is a response to stress. The child who wets his bed regularly may be a worrier. And of course, the greater the pressure he is under *not* to wet the bed the more the stress will grow—and the more likely he will be to wet his bed.

6. ECZEMA

Many mothers find it difficult to believe that anything as obvious and as real as an eczematous skin rash can possibly be caused by stress. And yet when you stop and think about it you will see that the skin is regularly affected by feelings and emotions. When we are frightened we go white. When we are angry we go red. When we are embarrassed we blush. Stress is by no means the only possible cause of an eczema rash. But whatever the basic cause of the rash may be, stress will almost always make things worse.

7. HEADACHES

There are other causes, of course, but most headaches are a result of stress, worry, anxiety and tension. If your child gets lots of headaches and the doctor can find no cause then take a look and see if he screws up his eyes when he is concentrating. If he gets a bad headache every evening after doing his homework you may be able to stop the headaches developing by teaching him to relax for a few minutes when he is half way through his work. Migraine headaches are often a result of stress too.

8. NAIL BITING

Children who are for ever nibbling their nails usually do so because they are anxious. The traditional, old fashioned remedy is to paint the nails with something that tastes horrid. This makes each nibble so revolting that the nails are eventually left alone. A slightly more modern remedy that works well with girls (and probably some boys) is to paint the nails with pretty coloured varnish. The theory is that the polish will make the recipient proud of her nails, more conscious of them and more determined not to bite them.

The trouble with both these techniques is that they only deal with the symptom and not the cause. Any child who bites his or her nails is over stressed. The problem will only be stopped for ever when the cause of the stress is dealt with.

9. SLEEPLESSNESS

When a child can't go to sleep there is often a simple explanation. The bedroom may be too hot or too cold. There may be too much noise. The child may not be tired. He may be in pain. But often children lie awake because they are anxious. They may be worried about problems at school or relationships at home—or they may be frightened because of something they have seen on television.

10. TICS, TWITCHES AND THUMB SUCKING

Tics are rapid, unexpected and repetitive movements which serve no purpose and which are entirely involuntary. They may involve the small muscles of the face and result in winking, blinking and simple twitching or they may involve larger muscles and produce coughing, sighing or shrugging. Whatever muscles they involve most are a result of stress, anxiety or tension. And the more a child worries about a tic the longer it will last.

When babies suck their thumbs it is natural and nothing

much to worry about. Young babies are born with a natural inclination to suck things which seem the right shape, size and texture. It is this inclination to suck which ensures that a baby takes to his mother's breast shortly after he is born. A baby's thumb, or indeed any of his fingers, is not all that different to a maternal nipple and thumb sucking is, therefore, a natural habit. Most children do it and most give up thumb sucking when they reach the age of three or four years old—without any parental intervention.

There are two things to watch out for. First, if a baby, infant or young child sucks his thumb a lot it might be a sign that he isn't getting enough love and attention. Or that he isn't getting long enough on the breast if he is being breast fed. If he is losing weight as well as sucking his thumb then he probably needs to spend more time sucking a nipple and less time sucking a thumb.

Second, thumb sucking may become a problem if it produces actual damage to the skin of the thumb or if it persists after the age of six. At that age it can push the teeth forward. Apart from these two things I suggest that you try to ignore thumb sucking. If you make too much fuss you could induce a feeling of anger and resentment in your child.

11. HEADBANGING

Babies often bang their heads for no apparent reason. As many as one in seven babies do it. Babies usually stop this rather worrying habit by themselves—though they may be three or four years old by the time they stop it. In the meantime try to make sure that there is nothing in her cot that your child can damage herself on (i.e. no sharp corners).

12. BREATH HOLDING

Breath holding attacks do not cause any physical damage. They simply result from a child's deliberate refusal to breathe and although they may sometimes follow pain or fear they are usually a result of the child feeling emotionally hurt, frustrated, thwarted or annoyed. Breath holding attacks are nothing more than very frightening, very effective temper tantrums. Children quickly learn to use them as a weapon to control their parents and to get their own way. They are very frightening but they aren't really dangerous. If your child holds his breath long enough he will eventually go unconscious and automatically start breathing again. The biggest real risk is that the shortage of oxygen to his brain may produce a convulsion.

There isn't a great deal you can do to abort a breath holding attack that has already started. The most important thing to remember is that you must try not to give in to the child who holds his breath in an attempt to force you to do something. I know it is difficult but try to stay calm. The more you panic—and the more he sees you panicking—the more he will use the trick to get his own way. Once your child learns that breath holding really doesn't pay he will soon give it up.

How you can help your child cope with stress

1   Try to decide whether or not your child is under too much stress. Could you be responsible? Do you push him too hard? Do you insist that he takes too much responsibility? Does he enjoy life or do you expect him to take life too seriously?

2   Look for early signs of stress. Does he get upset easily? Does he worry a lot about school? Does he seem very lonely? Does he get very upset if he doesn't do as well as expected in an examination or doesn't make a particular sports team? Is he always apologising?

3   If your child suffers from any particular symptoms—especially if they are persistent symptoms—ask yourself whether or not those symptoms could be caused or made worse by stress.

4   If you find him daydreaming don't tell him off. This is a simple, natural way of relaxing. There is nothing wrong with escaping from the real world for a few minutes occasionally.

5   Don't always expect him to be doing something useful.

6   Don't let your child get involved in too many stressful activ-

ities. If he is studying for examinations then he really should not be spending his free time on competitive sports. He needs a chance to relax at something that doesn't matter too much.

7 Try to spend some time each day just talking to him. Only by talking will you find out his worries. Like the rest of us children need to talk—and to feel that they can confide in someone they trust.

STROKE

About one in three of us will have a stroke—and one in seven of us will die of a stroke. Strokes are second only to heart attacks as a cause of death.

The commonest cause of a stroke is a blood clot. A clump of blood cells block one of the blood vessels supplying part of the brain. The result is that oxygen can't get through. The symptoms—paralysis and maybe a loss of speech—will depend on the area of the brain that is involved. Other causes of strokes include bleeding into the brain from a ruptured vessel.

Although strokes are a common cause of death they don't always kill. Indeed strokes are the commonest cause of disability in middle aged or elderly people.

Not surprisingly many people are terrified by the word 'stroke'—and imagine that all victims will be crippled for life. This simply isn't true. Every year, thousands of patients who have had strokes do recover, often through the love and encouragement of relatives and friends. Four out of five people who have strokes *do* learn to walk again.

Usually most of the recovery takes place in the first months or so—but improvement can continue after that for a year or more. The first two weeks are particularly important.

It's important to remember that a patient who can't talk and who seems unable to understand what is going on may understand and hear perfectly well. So never talk about a stroke victim as if he can't understand. Try to find out whether or not some form of conversation is possible—you may be able to converse by getting him to wiggle his fingers or flicker an eyelid.

STUTTERING

11 facts you should know

1   One in twenty people will stutter at some time in their lives.
2   At any one time the number of people stuttering will be around 1 in 100.
3   When children stutter it usually starts between the ages of 3 and 5.
4   Boys are affected more often than girls. As age increases stuttering becomes less and less common among girls.
5   Close relatives of stutterers are three times as likely to stutter as other members of the population.
6   There is a slight difference between stuttering and stammering. The stammerer speaks with hesitation. The stutterer has difficulty in speaking and also tends to repeat the first sounds of certain words.
7   There is no evidence that people who stutter have personality problems.
8   Stutterers and their parents are no more neurotic than anyone else.
9   It is not true that stuttering is caused by emotional trauma or problems in childhood.
10 Drugs, psychotherapy and hypnosis don't help. But regular work with a speech therapist can.
11 Some stutterers find they can help themselves by starting to speak as they breathe out.

SUICIDE

8 ways in which you can help prevent a suicide

1   Never ignore someone who talks of suicide. It is a *myth* that

people who talk of killing themselves never do it. Three out of four of those who kill themselves have talked about it beforehand—usually on several occasions.

2   Remember that those who have tried in the past are likely to try again in the future. And even if they bungled it so badly that it was dismissed as a 'cry for attention' there is a good chance that—either by accident or design—they will make a better job of it next time.

3   Learn to recognise the signs and symptoms of depression. If someone you know constantly apologises, frequently claims that he is a failure and never wants to go out then try to persuade him or her to talk. Show that you care. Remind him of his virtues and values. Make sure that medical advice is obtained.

4   Learn to share your love and your hopes and your friendship. Children—and especially teenagers—desperately need friendship.

5   Watch out for signs of deep depression—a loss of appetite, bursts of tears, sleeplessness. Once again—make sure that medical advice is obtained.

6   If you suspect that someone you know may try to commit suicide ask how desperate he feels. Get him to talk. Don't worry that you will be putting ideas into his head. That is unlikely. If he has thought about suicide he will probably know what you are getting at.

7   Clear out any unwanted pills in the medicine cabinet. If he is taking pills make sure that you take charge of the bottle.

8   Always get professional medical help if you suspect that someone you know is contemplating suicide.

TEETH

6 tips for looking after them

Dental decay is one of the commonest of all diseases. Dentists remove many tons of teeth every year and millions of children have mouths full of fillings. The two commonest of all tooth problems are gingivitis (an infection and inflammation of the gums) and dental caries (decaying teeth).

Gingivitis usually starts between the teeth or where the teeth meet the gums. The danger is that as the gums rot away so the teeth will become loose—and will eventually fall out.

Tooth decay occurs when the teeth are attacked by acids which are produced when bacteria in the mouth ferment sugar and food debris.

Both these problems can be avoided if teeth are looked after properly.

Follow this advice:

1   Don't eat too many sugary foods. Do not suck too many sugar rich sweets or sip too many sugary drinks.

2   Clean your teeth carefully at least once and preferably twice a day. It should take you five minutes to clean your teeth properly. Try to clean each tooth individually. You will spend between 3 and 6 months of your life brushing your teeth—you may as well learn how to do it properly.

3   Make sure that you have a new toothbrush regularly—probably once every three months. Buy a brush with bristles that feel soft to the touch. When the old brush is worn and the bristles are bent buy a new one. Press the bristles down with your finger—if they don't spring back into position then the brush should be 'retired' and used for cleaning the cooker.

4   Buy a toothpaste that contains fluoride. You can also get toothpastes that, in addition to containing fluoride, also help to control the production of tartar. Avoid abrasive powders.

5   Use dental floss to clean in between your teeth. Break off a length of floss, hold the two ends firmly in your two hands, and then insert the taut strand between your teeth. Pull it up and down to clear away the debris that would otherwise help rot your teeth.

6   Visit the dentist regularly for a check up. These days most modern dentists employ dental hygienists who can teach

you how to look after your teeth properly. Prevention is much better than treatment.

☞ *See also* Tooth problems.

TEETHING

Before we acquire our adult teeth we all have to acquire twenty milk teeth. These teeth see us through our early life until our jaws have developed and can accommodate the much larger teeth that will see us through adulthood.

The milk teeth appear during our first two or three years of life and their development is known as 'teething'.

Teething usually starts at about six months of age and continues until somewhere between 2 and 3. It is usually the teeth in the middle of the lower jaw that arrive first.

As the new teeth force their way through the gums they can sometimes produce a little pain—and there may be some redness and swelling of the gums too. The soreness and discomfort may occasionally make eating a little difficult and may interfere with sleep.

Plenty of myths exist about teething. I've heard it blamed for everything from asthma to worms—including fevers, diarrhoea, bronchitis, fits and skin rashes. But do try to ignore these myths. Teething is not a disease and it usually produces nothing more than teeth!

You can buy all sorts of tablets, powders, gels, creams and mixtures to help deal with the imagined problems said to be associated with teething. But I don't think any of these products are really worth buying.

You can, however, help teething in the following ways:

1 Give the child something hard to bite on. This may help relieve the discomfort and encourage teeth to erupt. A piece of hard food will do, but don't give a baby something it could swallow!

2 While teething children sometimes dribble. To prevent this irritating the skin put a little barrier cream onto the cheeks and chin.

3   Distract the child from any discomfort with a toy or a
    cuddle.

If you are worried or your child is in real pain, call your
doctor straight away. The chances are that it isn't teething that
is causing the problem.

Tetanus

Tetanus is an infection of the brain and spinal cord which is
caused by a bug called clostridium tetani—the spores of which
live mainly in fields and gardens.

The first symptom is stiffness of the jaw (known as lockjaw).
Other muscles then also become stiff. If the muscles of the chest
wall are affected the patient will have difficulty in breathing.
Children, gardeners and players of outdoor sports are particularly at risk. Tetanus can be prevented by regular
immunizations.

Thrush

How to avoid it and practical treatment tips

It won't kill you but it can make things pretty miserable. And
it can ruin your sex life.

Its proper name is candidiasis though its also known as monil-
iasis and its millions of sufferers know it as thrush.

And it is on the increase. Tens of thousands of women get it
for the first time every week. Hundreds of thousands—possibly
millions—are long term sufferers. Although it isn't necessarily
transmitted by sex (the fungus that causes it can just start to
grow) it often is and it's one of the commonest sexually transmitted diseases around.

If you haven't yet discovered the agonies of having thrush the
chances are that you will. The bug that causes the infection isn't
particularly rare. Most people have the candida albicans fungus
living on their skin or somewhere else in their bodies. But its
when the fungus starts to grow out of control that it causes
problems.

Theoretically the candida fungus can grow almost anywhere but like most fungi the infection that causes thrush prefers somewhere soft, moist, warm and dark. And that means that the vagina is the place most likely to be targeted.

The first symptom of thrush is usually a white, itchy discharge. Sex becomes painful, uncomfortable and unpleasant and the itching can be unbearable. Thick, white patches often appear around the outside of the vagina.

The chances of a candida fungal infection developing are increased when the naturally rather warm and moist area of the vagina is made unnaturally warmer or moister. Wearing nylon underwear, tights or close fitting trousers all make it easier for the candida fungus to grow.

But it isn't only what you wear that determines your susceptibility to thrush.

- The change in circulating oestrogens that occurs during pregnancy or when a woman takes the contraceptive pill can also encourage thrush to develop.
- Eating too much sugar makes the environment even better.
- Being overweight means that fatty folds around the outside of the vagina keep the area unusually moist and warm.
- Taking antibiotics upsets the natural balance of bugs and makes thrush more likely.
- Scratches and skin abrasions can also increase the likelihood of thrush developing.
- Inserting a tampon with dirty hands can also put up your chances of developing the infection.

There are many things you can do to reduce your chances of contracting thrush—or to increase your chances of getting rid of it.

1 Good local hygiene is important but it isn't necessary to use antiseptics or deodorants; indeed, such products can increase your problems by irritating the area.

2 Skirts, stockings and no underwear are much better for keeping the area well 'aired'.

3 Visit your doctor—he may prescribe an antifungal cream or pessaries. He may also want your partner to have a course

of treatment since infection can be passed between the two of you during sex.

4   Some women have reported a reduction in symptoms after dipping tampons in plain yoghurt and inserting them. Yoghurt contains the lactobacilli bacteria which compete with and often oust the infection.

TINNITUS

Tinnitus—or constant noises in the head or ears—can often be infuriating and distracting as well as deeply depressing. People have committed suicide because of tinnitus—it is a condition which is often underestimated by doctors. Patients deserve an enormous amount of sympathy and support though they often don't get much of either because there isn't anything much to see. The noises can vary from ringing to roaring and buzzing to hissing and whistling to clicking and they are only heard by the patient—others don't hear anything and so can't begin to comprehend the horrors of the disorder.

In tinnitus the acoustic nerve sends impulses to the brain not—as it should do—as a result of vibrations produced by external sound waves, but as a result of stimuli originating inside the head or even inside the ear itself. Patients who complain of tinnitus often also complain of some hearing loss. The causes include a condition called Meniere's disease, an infection of the inner ear (otitis media), andblockage of the outer canal with ear wax. Tinnitus can also be caused by damage to the ear, by a head injury or by some drugs—aspirin and quinine can cause it.

The noises heard may vary in type and intensity and although there is usually some noise there all the time the patient's perception of that noise may vary. Tolerance to the condition varies from one person to another.

Obviously, the first step is to try to decide whether or not there is an underlying problem that can be treated. If there is an infection, an injury or an inflammation then the appropriate therapy may lead to a fairly rapid improvement in the condition. When the tinnitus can't be removed some sufferers use headphones playing music to drown the noise—though this is not of course particularly satisfactory. Others get some relief from a tinnitus masker—headphones playing white noise, a random mixture of sounds of many different frequencies though this too isn't always entirely satisfactory.

Surgery has been tried for tinnitus but without particularly good results and a variety of drugs have been tried—again the results have varied. It is known that stress can make tinnitus worse and so it is also true that relaxation can make it better. Learning to relax won't cure tinnitus but it may make the symptoms less noticeable and more bearable.

My advice to anyone suffering from this condition is to make sure that you see an ear nose and throat surgeon, preferably one who takes a specialist interest in tinnitus—even if this means travelling away from your own area if there isn't a suitable consultant locally. A specialist should be able to find any curable underlying condition if there is one. And if there isn't then he should be able to offer some practical advice.

TIREDNESS

Causes and solutions

Buying a bottle of magic 'tonic' from your local chemist isn't necessarily the best answer for tiredness. Nearly half the patients who complain of tiredness are suffering from a specific, genuine physical problem. And most of the rest have a social or psychological problem.

If you are for ever feeling tired then you really should go and see your doctor and get a check up. A simple examination and a few blood tests may well provide the answer—and help your doctor solve the problem permanently.

Meanwhile, here is a list of some of the commonest causes of tiredness, together with other symptoms and possible treatments.

1. SLEEPLESSNESS

We recharge our batteries when we are asleep. If you are not sleeping properly then you're bound to feel tired. And sleeping pills aren't the answer—if taken for more than a couple of weeks they can cause sleeplessness. If you have difficulty in sleeping try this simple regime:

Walk for 10 minutes.

Think through your day's problems. Write down your worries in a notebook.

Spend 15 minutes in a soothing bath. Warm up your bed with a hot water bottle or electric blanket.

Go to bed with a relaxing book.

2. Poor eating habits

Your blood carries food and oxygen around your body. If your diet doesn't contain enough iron then your blood will be 'thin' and won't do its job properly. You can avoid this problem by eating plenty of fresh green vegetables. But if you think you could be anaemic, see your doctor.

3. Post viral fatigue syndrome

After a viral infection—such as flu or hepatitis—many people feel tired and washed out. Some people stay washed out for months. They may be suffering from 'post viral fatigue syndrome'—also known as myalgic encephalomyelitis (M.E.). This is especially common among men and women in their twenties and thirties. It causes mental and physical tiredness. Patients complain that they can't remember things and that they are clumsy and uncoordinated. There is no specific treatment but patients who rest when they are at their weakest will probably get better quicker.

4. Hormonal problems

Two specific hormone problems cause tiredness—diabetes and an underactive thyroid gland. Suspect diabetes if you feel thirsty, need to pass urine often, notice a weight change or suffer frequently from boils. Remember that diabetes runs in families.

Suspect thyroid problems if your other symptoms include poor memory, hoarse voice, thin hair, muscle cramps, poor appetite, weight gain, constipation, low sex drive and a hatred of cold weather.

Your doctor will be able to treat both these conditions effectively.

5. Overwork

If you work too hard—and constantly push yourself to your limits—you'll feed tired. The answer is obvious: you need to rest occasionally. And make sure that when you rest you really do rest. Try to get away completely every few months.

Tonsillitis

At the back of the mouth are two small lumps of lymph tissue known as the tonsils. These glands are intended to guard the air passageway and catch any infections which might try to enter the body. Under normal circumstances the tonsils do a difficult job extremely well. Problems arise when the tonsils are so badly infected and so filled with bacteria that their effectiveness is destroyed.

If the inflammation and infection of the tonsils persists then it is possible that your doctor will want the patient to have a tonsillectomy. Doctors now recognise that the tonsils perform a very useful role in the body's defences and usually only suggest removal as an act of last resort. No operation, however small, should be undertaken lightly or even considered until all the alternatives have been examined.

Removal of the tonsils only stops tonsillitis—it won't stop the patient getting sore throats.

Tooth problems

1. Toothache

Decayed teeth or irritated gums can be painful. The pain may come and go or may be continuous. When it is there it is usually throbbing. Hot or cold food may make it worse. Take paracetamol or soluble aspirin and try rinsing your mouth with warm or cold water (whichever helps most). Wrap a hot water bottle in a towel and hold it against your face (be careful not to burn your skin). Make an appointment to see a dentist as soon as possible—even if the pain disappears.

2. DENTAL ABSCESS

An abscess around a tooth causes persistent pain which is worse on biting and chewing. There will probably also be swelling and tenderness of the face and you may have foul taste in your mouth. Fix up an appointment to see your dentist or doctor urgently.

3. SOMETHING WEDGED BETWEEN THE TEETH

If you have a piece of food caught between your teeth try to dislodge it with a piece of dental floss or your toothbrush. Never use a hard, sharp or pointed instrument to try and clear the obstruction—there is a real risk that you will damage the tooth or gum. If you can't easily free the obstruction make an appointment with the dentist.

4. BROKEN OR CHIPPED TOOTH

Wash the broken tooth with warm water. Hold a cold compress to the side of the face to stop any swelling. Save the fragments of tooth if you can and take them to the dentist. He may be able to bond the fragments back into place. Never try gluing bits of tooth back into place yourself.

5. KNOCKED OUT TOOTH

If the tooth is dirty wash it in clean, running water. Hold the tooth by the top, not by the roots which are extremely delicate. Put the tooth into a container filled with water or wrap it in a damp cloth. Then get to the dentist's surgery as quickly as you can. If you get to your dentist quickly enough he may be able to replant the tooth—temporarily wiring it to neighbouring teeth to hold it in place.

6. MISSING FILLING

If you lose part of a filling make sure that you take special care to keep the tooth clean. Fix up an appointment to see the dentist as soon as possible.

7. DISCOLOURED TEETH

Teeth can be discoloured by:
- drinking lots of tea
- taking drugs (e.g. iron tablets)
- using some mouthwashes
- poor care

Your dentist can often remove or disguise the discoloration.

8. SENSITIVE TEETH

Sensitive teeth are very common—and the pain can be excruciating. Teeth become sensitive for two main reasons. First, if the gum recedes then tiny channels connecting the outside world to the nerve become exposed. It is normal for gums to recede with age (hence the phrase 'getting long in the tooth') but if your brushing is too energetic you may wear your gum away. Second, normal, healthy, young teeth are protected by a layer of enamel but too much over–energetic brushing can eventually wear this away—with the same sort of result.

When teeth are sensitive cold drinks and even cold weather can cause pain. Just brushing the teeth can lead to pain. Having 'sensitive' teeth may not sound like a serious problem but it can be: if you don't brush your teeth properly because they are too sensitive then you may easily develop tooth or gum disease. The best way to treat sensitive teeth is with a special type of tooth-paste. The proper toothpaste won't just help relieve the pain—it will also help cure the problem. If you are in any doubt about which to choose ask your dentist or pharmacist for advice.

☞ *See also* Bad breath; Teeth; Teething.

TRAVEL SICKNESS

6 tips to prevent it

Every summer thousands of holidays are ruined by travel sickness. The symptoms usually follow a predictable pattern. Patients start by feeling sweaty, nauseated and generally unwell. Heavy breathing, swallowing, yawning, drowsiness, pallor and vomiting follow.

I've lost count of the number of cures I've come across. Some parents advocate putting a chain on the back of the car. Others stick a piece of brown papers to the back of the child's shirt. Few of these home remedies work well.

The best way to avoid motion sickness is the persuade the potential sufferer to take an active interest in what is going on outside. In a car, for example, get your child to count lorries, look for blue cars, spot policemen—anything that involves him in the outside world. On a ship or aeroplane try to make sure that he can see outside.

Researchers have shown that when the brain is receiving plenty of information about what is going on outside the vehicle it balances that against the motion and is less likely to become disturbed.

This explains why car drivers are far less likely to suffer from motion sickness than passengers.

Here are some other useful tips.

1   Make sure that the sufferer doesn't eat anything too spicy, too rich or too fatty before travelling.

2   A snack while travelling will help.

3   If you want to try drugs ask the pharmacist for help.

4   Don't keep asking the sufferer if he feels nauseous.

5   Remember that although a third of all children suffer from motion sickness, many will grow out of it—usually after the age of ten.

6   Provide a sick bag to lessen the risk of panic.

ULCER

See Indigestion.

VARICOSE VEINS

Varicose veins are extremely common. About one in seven adults suffer from them. Women are more likely to have varicose veins than men. The disorder runs in families and tends to affect people who spend a good deal of their time standing still (for example hairdressers, dentists, shop assistants). Some varicose veins are painless—others cause an aching in the area, together with a swelling of the feet and ankles and some itching. The symptoms of varicose veins tend to get worse after the sufferer has been on her or his feet for a long period.

The symptoms are relieved by lying down or sitting down with the legs raised. Regular walking and wearing elastic support stockings will usually control most varicose veins but sometimes surgery is needed to deal with the problem.

VERRUCAE

Verrucae are infectious and are caused by the same virus that causes warts on the hands. 'Verruca' is the Latin name for a wart. Verrucae are flatter than other warts because they tend to get walked on. If you walked on your hands around your local swimming pool you could get verrucae on your hands though then they would be called warts. If you put your foot into the hand of someone with warts you could get a verruca. Children with verrucae should cover them up when swimming to reduce the chances of passing them on to other swimmers. All swimmers should wear plastic flip flop sandals when walking around the pool area, when in the changing room or when in the showers.

WARTS

Warts are small growths that are caused by a virus which stimulates the reproduction of skin cells. This can happen extremely quickly—warts can sometimes appear almost overnight!

Warts are infectious but there is still some controversy as to how easily they are transmitted.

Left alone most warts will disappear by themselves in about six months. This is little consolation to young adolescents who can find visible warts quite upsetting. Home remedies for treating warts can be bought from the pharmacy. Don't let children treat their own warts. Read the instructions carefully and make sure you only treat the wart—not the surrounding skin. Never try to surgically remove a wart.

You should always see a doctor if a wart changes colour, shape or size, or bleeds.

WEANING

8 facts you should know

1   Whether you are breast feeding or bottle feeding your baby will happily survive on milk for up to six to twelve months. Then you must start weaning. Do remember that the longer you can breast feed your baby the better. Many experts now believe that babies should be breast feed until they are close to their first birthday—because it is only then that they will have outgrown most of their food allergies.

2   Don't start weaning your baby off milk and on to solids too soon—if you do then you will run the risk of making him fat. A baby's intestines aren't ready to deal with solid food.

3   Tins of baby food are all right. But give your baby real, healthy food too. Give him a raw carrot or a stick of celery to chew on.

4   Don't add salt or sugar to a baby's meals.

5   Don't give your baby sweets or snacks between meals.

6   Most babies can start using spoons and cups at about six months of age. But expect a mess. It will probably be a year before he can handle them with any dexterity.

7   Don't get into battles over food. Surprisingly, babies and small children don't usually develop dietary deficiencies if they are allowed to choose their own food. But do see your doctor about any extreme fads or dislikes. And always see your doctor if you are worried about any aspects of your baby's diet.

8   A baby who has recurrent colic, vomiting, diarrhoea or

constipation is probably being overfed. The baby who fails to gain enough weight, draws up his legs in discomfort or who has difficulty in sleeping is probably being underfed.

☞ *See also* Baby feeding.

WHOOPING COUGH

Whooping cough is usually caused by an organism called bordetella pertussis and the infection is transmitted in droplets often coughed out by another victim of the disease. It tends to come in epidemics and is moderately common in childhood.

The incubation period is 1—2 weeks and the symptoms usually start like those of a cold with a runny nose and a cough. There is not usually a fever. The cough will gradually get worse and worse and after two or three weeks the characteristic 'whoop' will begin when the patient breathes in. There may also be some vomiting at this stage too. The coughing will often be worse at night.

Children with whooping cough should be kept away from school for four to six weeks and should be kept away from babies and older people. The disease can cause problems at both ends of the age spectrum—but particularly for babies. Get medical advice whenever you are concerned but always get urgent medical help when babies or young children have, or may have, the disease.

WIND

In adults

If you suffer from persistent or recurrent wind, you should, of course, go and see your doctor for personal advice. But if he is unable to help you and an examination shows no abnormality there may still be things that you can do to help yourself.

Here are some fairly simple to follow, straightforward tips designed to help you deal with wind both effectively and, I hope, permanently.

First, you should try to limit the amount of air that you

swallow. I know this probably sounds very obvious but two thirds of the gas in your body is probably swallowed air. You're likely to swallow too much air if you eat too quickly, gulp hot drinks or sip drinks through a straw. Habits like chewing gum and smoking can also cause wind to accumulate. Chewing with an open mouth or talking with your mouth full increase the likelihood of wind too.

Second, you should try to avoid the sort of foods that are likely to cause wind. Specific foods that are likely to cause problems include beans, broccoli, cabbage, raisins, bananas, popcorn, peanuts, onions, chocolate, coffee and milk. Fizzy drinks are an obvious cause. And although high fibre diets are very fashionable they can be a cause of wind in a lot of people so watch out—you may need to reduce your intake of fibre if you constantly suffer from wind. This may mean eating white bread instead of wholemeal bread, white pasta instead of wholemeal pasta and avoiding the skins of potatoes and other vegetables and fruits.

Third, make sure that you avoid getting constipated. Constipation does seem to be a common cause of wind. Make sure that you don't eat too many starchy, stodgy foods and do try to keep your fluid intake up: water and fruit juices are ideal.

Fourth, if the wind builds up try changing position—try sitting down, standing up, lying down or walking about. You might find that lying down in a warm bath helps.

Fifth, some sufferers find that sweets containing peppermint may help. Others swear by peppermint tea.

WIND

A special problem in babies

If you eat your meals with a knife and fork and drink out of a cup or glass the amount of air you swallow will be quite small. But if you try sucking up lots of liquid the chances are high that you will fill your stomach with air.

It is because they spend most of their feeding time sucking rather than chewing, drinking and swallowing that babies swallow so much air—and are so troubled by wind.

During the course of a single feeding session many babies will suck in enough air to form fairly large bubbles in their stomachs. The discomfort that occasionally results from this accumulation of wind isn't threatening in any way but it seems to worry parents a great deal.

There are many recommended remedies for wind. Sometimes special medicines are prescribed. On other occasions you will be told to get yourself and your baby into a position that would challenge a pair of professional contortionists.

The truth is that when a baby does acquire a bubble of wind in his stomach it is usually fairly easy to get rid of. You don't need to buy anything or make up any special medicine. And you don't need to wriggle into a difficult or uncomfortable position.

You simply have to remember that air will come up more easily when your baby is held upright. Lie a baby down when he has got wind in his stomach and the wind will be trapped where it is. But hold a baby upright and the wind will be able to escape from the stomach with ease. Rubbing or patting your baby on the back may give you something to do but I honestly don't think it will have much effect on the speed with which the air escapes. The vital factor is your baby's position—if he is upright then the wind will be able to get out.

Not all babies suffer from wind and there isn't anything you need to do if your baby always seems comfortable after feeding. On the other hand if your baby is a regular sufferer then you might be wise to hold him upright for a minute or two as a regular routine after every feed. It is much easier to deal with the potential problem before it develops than to have to pick up a baby who has been restless and uncomfortable and then try to get rid of the wind.

Since crying is the other common cause of wind, a baby who is uncomfortable and unhappy may well be adding fresh bubbles of air faster than the existing bubbles can be released. A nasty vicious circle can quickly develop.

It is important to know how to get rid of wind but it is even better to be able to stop it developing in the first place. Babies are by no means bound to suffer from accumulated air and when they do so there is often a reason for it.

It is no coincidence for example that the majority of babies who suffer from wind are those who are bottle fed. A baby who is breast feeding can wrap his lips quite tightly around his mother's nipple and as long as the milk is flowing freely there isn't too much chance of his sucking in air as well.

When a baby is feeding from a bottle, however, there are several ways in which air can get mixed up with the milk. First, and perhaps most important, it is vital to get the size of the hole in the bottle teat just right. If the hole is too small or too large then there is a real hazard of air getting in with the milk.

Next, it is important to make sure that the bottle is held at the correct angle. If a half empty bottle is held horizontally then there will be a good chance of your baby sucking in plenty of air, whatever the size of the teat. Make sure that the bottle is held as near to the vertical as seems possible.

Remember, too, that babies need to breathe as well as feed. If you don't allow your baby to have a break from the bottle occasionally then he will probably try sucking in air as he sucks at the bottle. That is almost bound to give him wind. When a baby has a cold and cannot breathe easily in through his nose this point is even more important.

Additionally, I think it is well worth remembering that whenever a baby brings up wind he is quite likely to bring up a little milk as well. This is natural and nothing to worry about.

As your baby's diet becomes more varied and he becomes mobile the problems with wind should diminish.

WINTER BLUES

7 ways to overcome it

Seasonal Affective Disorder (SAD) is a type of depression which affects people as the nights get longer and colder, the days get shorter, darker and gloomier and the weather forecasts get worse.

It is perhaps not surprising that enormous numbers of people regularly sink into a depression in the autumn from which they do not emerge until the blossom is back on the trees in the spring.

SAD isn't new. Hippocrates wrote about patients becoming depressed in the winter two thousand years ago.

But doctors have only recently realised just how serious SAD can be. And it has been established that it is a lack of light that is probably the main cause.

You could be a SAD sufferer if you answer YES to any of these simple questions during the winter months:

1   Do you feel tired and sleepy ?

2   Has your appetite increased—and have you started to put on weight?

3   Do you feel unwilling to go out in the evenings—but prefer to stay at home in front of the TV?

4   Do you binge on chocolate, biscuits and cake?

5   Do you have real difficulty in getting out of bed in the morning?

6   Are you losing interest in life?

If you have answered YES to any of these questions I suggest that you talk to your doctor. He may be able to offer specific treatment (such as helping you find a light box from which you can obtain artificial light treatment).

Here are some techniques you can use to help you defeat SAD this winter.

1   Eat a good breakfast—fruit juice, eggs, cereals, wholemeal bread, tea and coffee will all help. At lunchtime eat foods that give you energy but avoid alcohol. Have a very light snack in the evening.

2   Try to arrange your commitments so that you see some daylight every day—get up early or go outside at lunchtime if you work in an enclosed factory or office all day long.

3   If you feel tired in the daytime you may need to go to bed earlier—it's common to need more sleep in winter.

4   Get outdoors and exercise at weekends—a good walk will do you an enormous amount of good.

5   Make sure that light bulbs are powerful enough—the difference in price between a 100 watt light bulb and a 150 watt light bulb is very small.

6   Make sure you keep warm.

7   Try to plan a short winter break—it will be something to look forward to during the dark months ahead, particularly if you can afford somewhere sunny.

WORKAHOLISM

10 tips to help you survive

Workaholism—an unhealthy inability to stop working—is becoming commoner and commoner. It's usually caused by a long standing feeling of inadequacy. Some workaholics push themselves too hard because they are frightened of something: usually failure or poverty. But many simply feel the need to prove themselves better than anyone else.

If work is ruining your health it isn't too late to protect yourself.

First ask yourself these simple questions:

1   Are you always busy?

2   Do you feel constantly under pressure?

3   Do you wish you had more time for yourself?

4   Do you find it difficult to relax?

5   Are you unwilling to take a holiday—even though you need one?

6   Do you have difficulty in sleeping?

7   Do you work at evenings and weekends?

8   Do you snatch meals while you work?

9   Do you ever wake up at night thinking about work or money?

10 Do you find it difficult to slow your mind down?

If you have answered YES to any of these questions then you are almost certainly a workaholic.

Here are some of the diseases you could suffer from:

- Eczema or dermatitis
- Indigestion
- Irritable bowel syndrome
- Arthritis
- High blood pressure
- Asthma
- Headaches or migraines

You don't have to fit into particular working category to be a workaholic. People working for themselves often become victims as they struggle to create a successful business. But employees can also be victims—particularly if they are working in a tough, competitive environment with a ruthless and domineering boss. Housewives are as likely to suffer as anyone.

You can help yourself survive—in good health—by following some simple rules:

1   Cut out unnecessary work whenever possible. This is just as important at home as at work. Many chores become habits—even though they may not be necessary. Don't wash the car unless it's really dirty. Never iron socks or knickers.

2   Always leave a quarter of your time unscheduled. If you pack your day with appointments and commitments then the inevitable crises will throw you into a panic.

3   Make a list of everything you've got to do each week. Put urgent items on one list, less urgent items on a second list and non urgent items on a third list. This way you can make sure that you do the urgent stuff first—before you get chased.

4   Break down big jobs into small, manageable parts to reduce the stress levels.

5   If you have to take on something new try and make sure that you give up something that you are already doing—otherwise your work quota will simply expand until you collapse.

6 Allow other people to help you as often as possible. At work delegate whenever you can. Try to surround yourself with people whom you can trust. At home, when they are old enough, get the kids to help with the washing up and peel the potatoes; then, gradually increase their responsibilities.

7 Make relaxation a priority—and put it on your *urgent* list every week. You should spend some time every day relaxing—and you need to be able to relax effectively and thoroughly.

8 Make physical fitness a priority—put visits to the gym on your *urgent* list too. The fitter you are the better you will be able to cope with stress and pressure.

9 Don't let your work invade every aspect of your life. If you take work home make sure that you only work in *one* room.

10 Learn to say 'no'. It may be hard. But it is often a lot easier than saying 'yes' to things that you don't really want to do, and haven't got time for.

Finally, don't make the mistake of thinking that you are indispensable. Graveyards are full of people who thought they were indispensable.

If you want to know just how indispensable you are try this:
● Fill a bowl with warm water;
● Put your hand into the bowl;
● Take your hand out;
● Now look at the size of the hole your hand leaves when you remove it.

That's how indispensable you are.

WORMS

There are many types of parasitic worms which affect humans.

Threadworms are said to be present in one in three children. They look like tiny cotton threads and are about one centimetre long. The worms breed in the intestines and the eggs are passed in the stools. They can cause itching, and if the sufferer scratches he may pick up the eggs on his hands and transfer them back into the intestines.

Roundworms look like ordinary garden earthworms. You catch them by swallowing an egg which hatches in the intestine. The larva then burrows through the intestinal wall, enters a vein and is carried to the heart and then into the lungs. In the lungs the larva causes an infection which produces a cough—it is brought up with the sputum and swallowed so that it gets back into the intestine. There it develops into an adult worm.

Tapeworms can measure several metres long and look like a piece of long ribbon. They have a very complicated life cycle with the adults living in humans and the eggs living in another host such as a pig or cow.

Toxocara are worms which usually live in cats or dogs. They spread to humans through the faeces of the animal concerned. The larvae of these worms can move into the liver, the central nervous system and the eyes. They can cause very serious damage and an infection with toxocara worms can lead to blindness.

Worms are usually infectious and children tend to be most at risk. Ensure that they wash their hands after every visit to the lavatory. If you have a pet cat or dog make sure that the animal is regularly examined and wormed.

See your doctor for the treatment of worms.

WRINKLES

Wrinkles are an inevitable consequence of growing old. As we get older so the connective tissue beneath the skin loses its firmness, the elastic fibres break down, the skin loses its natural plasticity and changes in sex hormone production alter the quantities of skin oils being produced.

All these factors combine with environmental hazards—such as sunshine, high winds and chemical pollutants—to produce wrinkling.

Apart from plastic surgery there really isn't any way to make wrinkles disappear. You can cover up wrinkles with creams. But I don't think either massage or exercise will make wrinkles disappear.

The best way to protect your skin from wrinkling is to use a moisturising cream regularly and to avoid spending too much time in the sun. Keeping away from cigarette smoke will also help since smoke makes most people screw up their eyes—and that causes wrinkles.

Appendix 1

HOW MUCH SHOULD YOU WEIGH?

Height/weight chart for women

Instructions
1. Weigh yourself with as few clothes as possible—and no shoes
2. Measure your height in bare or stockinged feet
3. You are overweight if your weight falls above your ideal weight band

Height (feet & inches)	Ideal Weight Band (stones & pounds)
4.10	7.5—8.5
4.11	7.7—8.7
5.0	7.9—8.9
5.1	7.11—8.11
5.2	8.1—9.1
5.3	8.4—9.4
5.4	8.6—9.6
5.5	8.10—9.10
5.6	9.0—10.0
5.7	9.3—10.3
5.8	9.7—10.7
5.9	9.10—10.10
5.10	10.0—11.0
5.11	10.3—11.3
6.0	10.7—11.7
6.1	10.9—11.9
6.2	10.12—11.12
6.3	11.2—12.2
6.4	11.5—12.5

Note Ideal weights vary with age and various other factors. But if you weigh more than 14 pounds above the maximum in your Ideal Weight Band then your weight will almost certainly be having an adverse effect on your health.

Height/weight chart for men

Instructions
1. Weigh yourself with as few clothes as possible—and no shoes
2. Measure your height in bare feet
3. You are overweight if your weight falls above your Ideal Weight Band

Height (feet & inches)	Ideal Weight Band (stones & pounds)
5.0	8.5—9.5
5.1	8.6—9.6
5.2	8.7—9.7
5.3	8.8—9.8
5.4	8.11—9.11
5.5	9.2—10.2
5.6	9.6—10.6
5.7	9.10—10.10
5.8	10.0—11.0
5.9	10.4—11.4
5.10	10.8—11.8
5.11	10.12—11.12
6.0	11.2—12.2
6.1	11.6—12.6
6.2	11.10—12.10
6.3	12.0—13.0
6.4	12.4—13.4
6.5	12.8—13.8
6.6	13.0—14.0

Note Ideal weights vary with age and various other factors. But if you weigh more than 14 pounds above the maximum in your Ideal Weight Band, your weight will almost certainly be having an adverse effect on your health.

Appendix 2

AVERAGE HEIGHT AND WEIGHT TABLES FOR CHILDREN

Parents often worry about whether or not their children are tall enough, fat enough, thin enough or too tall, too fat or too thin! Subjective assessments are of little value. The tables which follow are intended to provide a rough and ready guide to the range within which normal healthy children may reasonably be expected to fall. Average heights and weights (for what they are worth) can be estimated by simply finding the figure in the middle of the two extremes I have quoted.

Average height and weight

Girls

Age	Weight (lbs)	Length/Height(ins)
3 months	9–15	21–24
6 months	13–21	24–27
1 year	17–26	27–31
2 years	21–33	31–36
3 years	26–41	34–39
4 years	29–45	36–41
5 years	32–50	39–46
6 years	35–56	41–49
7 years	40–62	43–51
8 years	43–69	45–54
9 years	47–77	47–56
10 years	51–85	49–59
11 years	55–105	51–61
12 years	61–115	52–63
14 years	80–135	57–67
16 years	95–155	59–68

Boys

Age	Weight(lbs)	Length/height (ins)
3 months	9–15	22–25
6 months	14–22	24–28
1 year	19–28	28–32
2 years	22–34	32–37
3 years	26–39	34–41
4 years	29–44	37–43
5 years	32–50	40–46
6 years	36–55	41–48
7 years	39–63	43–51
8 years	42–70	45–53
9 years	46–80	47–56
10 years	50–89	48–58
11 years	55–97	51–60
12 years	63–108	52–63
14 years	75–135	56–68
16 years	95–155	61–73

Appendix 3

YOUR MEDICAL RECORDS

Can you remember whether you have had measles, mumps or chickenpox? Are you allergic to any drugs? Can you remember the names? Can you remember whether you have had a tetanus jab?

You probably can't! So why not start keeping your own medical records *now*. You'll find it useful—and your children will be grateful when they grow up and want to know what they have or haven't had. You may think now that you'll never forget those first spots or vaccinations—but you will forget the dates!

The medical records that your doctor keeps aren't always as complete as they should be. And they often are not available. This absence of information can make life tricky when you are away from home or filling in a form. And in an emergency not knowing something could be life threatening.

Name _____

Disease/date

_____
_____
_____
_____
_____
_____
_____
_____

Vaccination/date

_____
_____
_____
_____

Allergy/date

_____
_____
_____

Notes

Name _____

Disease/date

_____
_____
_____
_____
_____
_____
_____
_____

Vaccination/date

_____
_____
_____
_____
_____

Allergy/date

_____ .
_____
_____
_____

Notes

Name _____

Disease/date

_____
_____
_____
_____
_____
_____
_____
_____

Vaccination/date

_____
_____
_____
_____
_____

Allergy/date

_____
_____
_____
_____

Notes

Name _____

Disease/date

_____
_____
_____
_____
_____
_____
_____
_____

Vaccination/date

_____
_____
_____
_____

Allergy/date

_____
_____
_____

Notes

Name _____

Disease/date

_____
_____
_____
_____
_____
_____
_____

Vaccination/date

_____
_____
_____
_____

Allergy/date

_____
_____
_____

Notes

Also published by the European Medical Journal

Relief from IBS

Simple steps for long-term control

Vernon Coleman

- Causes and symptoms of Irritable Bowel Syndrome
- The two-step control programme
- How you should change your diet
- How to look after your digestive system
- Relief from wind
- Watch out for foods that make your symptoms worse
- Stand up for yourself
- Build up your self-confidence
- Learn to relax your body and mind
- How worrying more can help you worry less
- Tips to help you cope with stress
- Take control of your life

1 898947 03 1
128pp   paperback   £9.95

Available from Book Sales, Publishing House,
Trinity Place, Barnstaple, Devon EX32 9HJ, England.
Please write for a catalogue.

Also published by the European Medical Journal

Why Animal Experiments Must Stop
And how you can help stop them
Vernon Coleman

"The most damning indictment of vivisection
ever published"

"Essential reading for anyone wishing to counter the
arguments of the vivisectors"

Dr Coleman analyses all the pro-vivisection arguments one by one—and destroys them. The moral, ethical, scientific and medical arguments are all dealt with.

Animal tests can produce dangerously misleading information. Penicillin kills cats and guinea pigs. Aspirin kills cats. Digitalis is so toxic to animals that it would never have been cleared for humans, but it remains our most useful heart drug. Yet practolol, which was judged safe after animal tests, caused damage to human patients and had to be withdrawn.

Dr Coleman makes it clear that animal experiments are useless today and have always been useless.

This book also describes the alternatives to animal experiments. It offers readers a 10-point plan to help them make sure that vivisection is stopped, putting an end to one of the world's most barbaric practices.

ISBN 0 9521492 1 4
128pp paperback £9.95

Available from Book Sales, Publishing House,
Trinity Place, Barnstaple, Devon EX32 9HJ, England.
Please write for a catalogue.

Food for Thought
Your guide to healthy eating
Vernon Coleman

Packed with easy-to-use, up to date, practical information, *Food for Thought* is designed to help you differentiate between fact and fantasy when planning your diet. The book's 28 chapters include:

- Food the fuel: basic information about carbohydrates, protein, fat, vitamins and minerals
- When water isn't safe to drink—and what to do about it
- How what you eat affects your health
- Why snacking is good for you
- The mini-meal diet and the painless way to lose weight
- Quick tips for losing weight
- The Thirty-Nine Steps to Slenderness
- 20 magic superfoods that can improve your health
- The harm food additives can do
- 20-point plan for avoiding food poisoning
- Drugs and hormones in food
- Food irradiation, genetically altered food, microwaves
- 30 common diseases—and their relationship to what you eat
- How to eat a healthy diet
- 21 reasons for being a vegetarian
- How much should you weigh?
- How to deal with children who are overweight

ISBN 0 9521492 6 5 192pp paperback £9.95

Available from Book Sales, Publishing House, Trinity Place, Barnstaple, Devon EX32 9HJ, England. Please write for a catalogue.

Betrayal of Trust

Vernon Coleman

Betrayal of Trust follows in the tradition of Vernon Coleman's most iconoclastic and ground-breaking books—*The Medicine Men, Paper Doctors,* and *The Health Scandal.*

Dr Coleman catalogues the incompetence and dishonesty of the medical profession and the pharmaceutical industry and explains the historical background to the problems which exist today. He shows how drugs are put onto the market without being properly tested, and provides hard evidence for his astonishing assertion that doctors now do more harm than good.

To support his claim that drug companies use animal tests to get their drugs on the market, Dr Coleman lists scores of widely prescribed drugs which are reguarly prescribed for patients, despite the fact that there is evidence showing that the drugs cause serious problems when given to animals.

Drug companies are, he explains, in a 'no lose' situation. If a new drug seems safe when given to animals, the company making it uses that evidence to help get the drug a licence. But if a new drug causes problems when given to animals, that evidence is ignored as irrelevant! Only patients lose.

"When animal experiments are stopped," says Dr Coleman, "they will never be reintroduced. The moral, ethical, scientific and medical evidence all supports the contention than animal experiments must be stopped now."

ISBN 0 9521492 2 2 160pp £9.95

Available from Book Sales, Publishing House,
Trinity Place, Barnstaple, Devon EX32 9HJ, England.
Please write for a catalogue.

Also published by the European Medical Journal

How to Conquer Pain

A new and positive approach to the problem of persistent and recurrent pain

Vernon Coleman

A fully revised and updated edition of *Natural Pain Control.*

This book tells you
- Factors which influence the amount of pain you feel
- Doctors, drugs and pain control
- How to get the best out of pills
- Alternative therapies that work
- The unique Pain Control Progamme
- How to use your imagination to conquer your pain
- How to sleep when pain is the problem
- The magic of the TENS machine
- Learn how to relax and control your stress
- How to measure your pain
- •• and lots, lots more! ••

What they said about the first edition:
☞ A clear and helpful handbook for pain sufferers... Perhaps most important of all is the way in which it brings pain down to a manageable level and gives self help ideas for sufferers.
The Guardian
☞ Full of good ideas *Mother and Baby*
☞ A new and positive approach *Keep Fit*
☞ An authoritative guide to this universal problem
Bournemouth Evening Echo

ISBN 0 9521492 9 X   192pp paperback £9.95

Available from Book Sales, Publishing House,
Trinity Place, Barnstaple, Devon EX32 9HJ, England.
Please write for a catalogue.

Also published by the European Medical Journal

Bodypower
The secret of self-healing
Vernon Coleman

A new edition of a book that hit the *Sunday Times* and *Bookseller* 'Top Ten' charts.

- How your body can heal itself
- How your personality affects your health
- How to use bodypower to stay healthy
- How to stay slim for life
- How to conquer 90% of all illnesses without a doctor
- How to improve your eyesight
- How to fight cancer
- How to use bodypower to help you break bad habits
- How to relax your body and your mind
- How to use bodypower to improve your shape
- •• and much, much more! ••

What they said about the first edition:
☞ Don't miss it! Dr Coleman's theories could change your life
Sunday Mirror
☞ If you've got Bodypower, you may never need visit your doctor again, or take another pill! *Slimmer*
☞ A marvellously succint and simple account of how the body can heal itself without resort to drugs *Spectator*
☞ Could make stress a thing of the past *Woman's World*
☞ Shows you how to listen to your body *Woman's Own*
☞ Could help save the NHS from slow strangulation
The Scotsman

ISBN 0 9521492 8 1   192pp   paperback   £9.95

Available from Book Sales, Publishing House,
Trinity Place, Barnstaple, Devon EX32 9HJ, England.
Please write for a catalogue.

Also published by the European Medical Journal

Mindpower

How to use your mind to heal your body

Vernon Coleman

The first edition of this book hit the *Sunday Times* and
Bookseller 'Top Ten' charts.

- A new approach to health care
- How your mind influences your body
- How to control destructive emotions
- How to deal with guilt
- How to harness positive emotions
- How daydreaming can relax your mind
- How to use your personal strengths
- How to conquer your weaknesses
- How to teach yourself mental self defence
- Specific advice to help you enjoy good health
- •• and much, much more! ••

What they said about the first edition:
☞ Dr Coleman explains the importance of a patient's mental
attitude in controlling and treating illness, and suggests some
easy-to-learn techniques *Woman's World*
☞ An insight into the most powerful healing agent in the
world—the power of the mind *Birmingham Post*
☞ Based on an inspiring message of hope *Western Morning
News*
☞ It will be another bestseller *Nursing Times*

ISBN 1 898947 00 7   192pp   paperback   £9.95

Available from Book Sales, Publishing House,
Trinity Place, Barnstaple, Devon EX32 9HJ, England.
Please write for a catalogue.